Ophthalmology: New Diagnostic and Treatment Approaches

Ophthalmology: New Diagnostic and Treatment Approaches

Guest Editors

Stephen G. Schwartz
Krishna S. Kishor
Víctor M. Villegas
Christopher Leffler
Andrzej Grzybowski

MDPI

Basel • Beijing • Wuhan • Barcelona • Belgrade • Novi Sad • Cluj • Manchester

Guest Editors
Stephen G. Schwartz
Bascom Palmer Eye Institute
University of Miami Miller
School of Medicine
Naples, FL
USA

Krishna S. Kishor
Bascom Palmer Eye Institute
University of Miami Miller
School of Medicine
Palm Beach Gardens, FL
USA

Víctor M. Villegas
Department of
Ophthalmology
University of Puerto Rico
School of Medicine
San Juan, PR
USA

Christopher Leffler
Department of
Ophthalmology
Virginia Commonwealth
University
Richmond, VA
USA

Andrzej Grzybowski
Institute for Research in
Ophthalmology
Foundation for
Ophthalmology Development
Poznan
Poland

Editorial Office
MDPI AG
Grosspeteranlage 5
4052 Basel, Switzerland

This is a reprint of the Special Issue, published open access by the journal *Medicina* (ISSN 1648-9144), freely accessible at: https://www.mdpi.com/journal/medicina/special_issues/374PR2P11D.

For citation purposes, cite each article independently as indicated on the article page online and as indicated below:

Lastname, A.A.; Lastname, B.B. Article Title. *Journal Name* **Year**, *Volume Number*, Page Range.

ISBN 978-3-7258-5581-0 (Hbk)
ISBN 978-3-7258-5582-7 (PDF)
https://doi.org/10.3390/books978-3-7258-5582-7

Contents

medicina

MDPI

Editorial

Editorial for Special Issue "Ophthalmology: New Diagnostic and Treatment Approaches"

Stephen G. Schwartz [1,*], Krishna S. Kishor [2], Victor M. Villegas [3], Christopher T. Leffler [4] and Andrzej Grzybowski [5]

1 Department of Ophthalmology, Bascom Palmer Eye Institute, University of Miami Miller School of Medicine, Naples, FL 34103, USA
2 Department of Ophthalmology, Bascom Palmer Eye Institute, University of Miami Miller School of Medicine, Palm Beach Gardens, FL 33418, USA; kkishor@med.miami.edu
3 Department of Ophthalmology, University of Puerto Rico School of Medicine, San Juan, PR 00936, USA; victor.villegas@upr.edu
4 Department of Ophthalmology, Virginia Commonwealth University School of Medicine, Richmond, VA 23298, USA; chrisleffler md@gmail.com
5 Foundation for Ophthalmology Development, 61-836 Poznan, Poland; ae.grzybowski@gmail.com
* Correspondence: sschwartz2@med.miami.edu

Introduction

There have been many recent advances in the diagnosis and treatment of eye diseases. The aim of this Special Issue is to publish new evidence and to review the current state-of-the-art developments in the diagnosis and treatment of vision-threatening diseases. This Special Issue features nine original contributions, including basic science investigations, clinical studies, and review articles.

Ichikawa and colleagues [1] investigated fibronectin adhesion to three types of intraocular lenses (IOLs): collamer-based EVO + Visian implantable contact lenses (ICLs); hydrophilic acrylic implantable phakic contact lens (IPCLs); and hydrophilic acrylic phakic-IOLs (LENTIS) used as controls. Under the experimental conditions studied, minimal fibronectin deposition and cellular adhesion was noted in the central optical zone of all three IOLs. However, the haptics of the collamer IOLs developed a thin fibronectin film. The investigators concluded that the collamer IOLs may promote fibronectin film formation, which may affect long-term transparency and biocompatibility.

Bartusis and colleagues [2] conducted a cross-sectional observational study comparing intracranial pulse wave signals in patients with normal-tension glaucoma (NTG) and age-matched controls. The investigators reported that median intracranial pulse wave amplitude was significantly higher in patients with NTG, which suggests that this noninvasive screening device may serve as a potential biomarker for this difficult-to-diagnose condition.

Sicks and colleagues [3] irradiated porcine and human corneas using 222 nm Far-UVC and reported that treatment with up to 60 mJ/cm^2 did not significantly affect corneal cell integrity and caused only a 3.7% reduction in cell density. The investigators proposed that irradiation under these conditions may be effective in decontaminating donor corneas, thus increasing the available supply of tissue for surgical patients.

Otake and colleagues [4] studied the effects of increasing ambient temperature on human lens epithelial cells. Using shotgun liquid chromatography with tandem mass spectrometry-based global proteomics, they reported differences in proteins digested from the immortalized human lens epithelial cell line iHLEC-NY2 at normal (35 degrees C) and warming (37.5 degrees C) temperatures. They proposed that differences in protein expression under warming conditions may contribute to the pathogenesis of cataract development.

Chen and colleagues [5] applied Shapley additive explanation (SHAP) techniques with machine learning to review intraocular pressure changes among pediatric patients treated with atropine to slow myopia progression. The investigators proposed that this approach may improve our ability to make more personalized treatment decisions for these patients.

Murati Calderón and colleagues [6] reviewed emerging therapies for retinitis pigmentosa. Voretigene neparvovec is approved for the treatment of patients with *RPE65*-associated disease. Gene-based therapeutic strategies currently being investigated include gene replacement therapies, gene editing using CRISPR-Cas9, RNA-based therapies, and optogenetic therapies.

Ruiz-Justiz and colleagues [7] presented current practices for the surgical care of pediatric patients requiring combined cataract surgery and pars plana vitrectomy. This approach is generally used for patients with congenital cataracts, ectopia lentis, retinopathy of prematurity, retinal detachment, and persistent fetal vasculature. The advantages and disadvantages of lens-sparing vitrectomy versus combined surgery are discussed.

Rosado and colleagues [8] surveyed the pathogenesis and management of Bardet-Biedl syndrome. Clinical manifestations include retinal degeneration, corneal abnormalities, strabismus, nystagmus, cataracts, and optic nerve abnormalities. Investigational therapies include gene replacement therapies, gene-editing using CRISPR-Cas9, nonsense suppression (readthrough) therapy, and neuroprotective therapies.

Olawade and colleagues [9] reviewed applications of artificial intelligence to ophthalmology, including machine learning and deep learning techniques. The investigators report that artificial intelligence may improve diagnostic accuracy and personalized treatment plans for patients with ophthalmic diseases.

We believe that these nine contributions improve our current understanding of ophthalmology and have the potential to stimulate further research.

Author Contributions: Writing—original draft preparation, S.G.S.; writing—review and editing, K.S.K., V.M.V., C.T.L. and A.G. All authors have read and agreed to the published version of the manuscript.

Funding: This research was partially supported by Research to Prevent Blindness—Unrestricted Grant GR004596-1 to the University of Miami.

Conflicts of Interest: The authors declare no conflicts of interest. The funders had no role in the design of the study; in the collection, analyses, or interpretation of data; in the writing of the manuscript; or in the decision to publish the results.

References

1. Ichikawa, K.; Tanaka, Y.; Horai, R.; Kato, Y.; Ichikawa, K.; Yamamoto, N. Comparison of Adhesion of Immortalized Human Iris-Derived Cells and Fibronectin on Phakic Intraocular Lenses Made of Different Polymer Base Materials. *Medicina* **2025**, *61*, 1384. [CrossRef]
2. Bartusis, L.; Krakauskaite, S.; Kevalaite, U.; Judickaite, A.; Zizas, A.; Stoskuviene, A.; Chaleckas, E.; Deimantavicius, M.; Hamarat, Y.; Scalzo, F.; et al. Non-invasive Monitoring of Intracranial Pressure Pulse Waves from Closed Eyelids in Patients with Normal-Tension Glaucoma. *Medicina* **2025**, *61*, 566. [CrossRef] [PubMed]
3. Sicks, B.; Hessling, M.; Stucke-Straub, K.; Kupferschmid, S.; Lotfi, R. Disinfection of Human and Porcine Corneal Endothelial Cells by Far-UVC Irradiation. *Medicina* **2025**, *61*, 416. [CrossRef] [PubMed]
4. Otake, H.; Yamamoto, T.; Yamamoto, N.; Nakazawa, Y.; Miyata, Y.; Taga, A.; Sasaki, H.; Nagai, N. Changes in Protein Expression in Warmed Human Lens Epithelium Cells Using Shotgun Proteomics. *Medicina* **2025**, *61*, 286. [CrossRef] [PubMed]
5. Chen, J.-W.; Chen, H.-A.; Liu, T.-C.; Wu, T.-E.; Lu, C.-J. The Potential of SHAP and Machine Learning for Personalized Explanations of Influencing Factors in Myopic Treatment for Children. *Medicina* **2025**, *61*, 16. [CrossRef] [PubMed]

6. Murati Calderón, R.A.; Emanuelli, A.; Izquierdo, N. Retinitis Pigmentosa: From Genetic Insights to Innovative Therapeutic Approaches—A Literature Review. *Medicina* **2025**, *61*, 1179. [CrossRef] [PubMed]
7. Ruiz-Justiz, A.J.; Cruz-Villegas, V.; Schwartz, S.G.; Villegas, V.M.; Murray, T.G. Combined Cataract and Vitrectomy Surgery in Pediatric Patients. *Medicina* **2025**, *61*, 1176. [CrossRef] [PubMed]
8. Rosado, A.; Rodriguez, E.; Izquierdo, N. Ophthalmologic Manifestations in Bardet-Biedl Syndrome: Emerging Therapeutic Approaches. *Medicina* **2025**, *61*, 1135. [CrossRef] [PubMed]
9. Olawade, D.B.; Weerasinghe, K.; Mathugamage, M.D.D.E.; Odetayo, A.; Aderinto, N.; Teke, J.; Boussios, S. Enhancing Ophthalmic Diagnosis and Treatment with Artificial Intelligence. *Medicina* **2025**, *61*, 433. [CrossRef] [PubMed]

medicina

MDPI

Article

The Potential of SHAP and Machine Learning for Personalized Explanations of Influencing Factors in Myopic Treatment for Children

Jun-Wei Chen [1], Hsin-An Chen [1], Tzu-Chi Liu [2], Tzu-En Wu [3,4] and Chi-Jie Lu [2,5,6,*]

1 School of Medicine, Chang Gung University, Taoyuan 333, Taiwan
2 Graduate Institute of Business Administration, Fu Jen Catholic University, New Taipei City 242, Taiwan
3 School of Medicine, Fu Jen Catholic University, New Taipei City 242, Taiwan
4 Department of Ophthalmology, Shin Kong Wu Ho-Su Memorial Hospital, Taipei 111, Taiwan
5 Artificial Intelligence Development Center, Fu Jen Catholic University, New Taipei City 242, Taiwan
6 Department of Information Management, Fu Jen Catholic University, New Taipei City 242, Taiwan
* Correspondence: 059099@mail.fju.edu.tw; Tel.: +886-2-29052973

Abstract: *Background and Objectives:* The rising prevalence of myopia is a significant global health concern. Atropine eye drops are commonly used to slow myopia progression in children, but their long-term use raises concern about intraocular pressure (IOP). This study uses SHapley Additive exPlanations (SHAP) to improve the interpretability of machine learning (ML) model predicting end IOP, offering clinicians explainable insights for personalized patient management. *Materials and Methods:* This retrospective study analyzed data from 1191 individual eyes of 639 boys and 552 girls with myopia treated with atropine. The average age of the whole group was 10.6 ± 2.5 years old. The refractive error of spherical equivalent (SE) in myopia degree was base SE at 2.63D and end SE at 3.12D. Data were collected from clinical records, including demographic information, IOP measurements, and atropine treatment details. The patients were divided into two subgroups based on a baseline IOP of 14 mmHg. ML models, including Lasso, CART, XGB, and RF, were developed to predict the end IOP value. Then, the best-performing model was further interpreted using SHAP values. The SHAP module created a personalized and dynamic graphic to illustrate how various factors (e.g., age, sex, cumulative duration, and dosage of atropine treatment) affect the end IOP. *Results*: RF showed the best performance, with superior error metrics in both subgroups. The interpretation of RF with SHAP revealed that age and the recruitment duration of atropine consistently influenced IOP across subgroups, while other variables had varying effects. SHAP values also offer insights, helping clinicians understand how different factors contribute to predicted IOP value in individual children. *Conclusions:* SHAP provides an alternative approach to understand the factors affecting IOP in children with myopia treated with atropine. Its enhanced interpretability helps clinicians make informed decisions, improving the safety and efficacy of myopia management. This study demonstrates the potential of combining SHAP with ML models for personalized care in ophthalmology.

Keywords: myopia; atropine; intraocular pressure; machine learning; SHAP value

1. Introduction

Myopia severity has increased globally, becoming a major concern for ophthalmologists. Currently, it affects 1.4 billion people (22.9% of the population) and is expected to affect 4.8 billion people (49.8%) by 2050 [1]. Studies link myopia incidence to race and other risk factors, with rates rising in both Western and Asian countries [2,3], especially among younger Asian women, according to some studies [4].

Clinicians are focused on controlling myopia progression, with three main treatments for adolescents, namely atropine eye drops, orthokeratology (OK) lenses, and peripheral defocus spectacle lenses [5,6]. These interventions aim to decelerate myopia progression and reduce the risk of associated complications, such as cataracts, retinal detachment, optic atrophy, glaucoma, retinal detachment, chorioretinal atrophy, and lacquer cracks. These conditions can lead to irreversible visual impairment and severe sequelae, leading to blindness.

Atropine effectively controls myopia progression and prevents high myopia [7,8]. However, concerns about the side effects of long-term usage have grown among parents and clinicians [9]. Atropine, a non-selective antimuscarinic agent with high affinity for M1–M5 receptors, causes mydriasis and cycloplegia in the pupillary sphincter ciliary muscle. Common reported side effects of topical atropine include light sensitivity, blurred near vision due to pupil dilation, and temporary accommodation [10,11]. Additionally, atropine may increase resistance through the trabecular meshwork, potentially impeding aqueous humor flow into the Schlemm's canal [12]. Pupillary dilation has been identified as a predisposing factor for glaucoma [13]. Atropine and other anticholinergic agents may elevate intraocular pressure (IOP), making them contraindicated in patients with glaucoma [14]. In normal children, IOP gradually increases with age, stabilizing at adult levels around age 12 [15]. The safety of this treatment remains a subject of ongoing debate, particularly regarding its potential to elevate intraocular pressure (IOP). It is well established that individuals with myopia are at a higher risk of developing glaucoma, including normotensive glaucoma. Consequently, there is significant clinical interest in establishing reliable prognostic factors to identify contraindications or limitations for atropine use in patients at risk of increased IOP.

Previous studies employing biostatistical methods have conducted retrospective or prospective studies on children with myopia treated with atropine, indicating that atropine treatment does not pose a high risk of IOP exceeding safety thresholds that could lead to glaucoma [16]. Furthermore, machine learning (ML) analyzed the data by extreme gradient boosting (XGB) and found that base IOP was the most influential factor affecting the final IOP [17]. Moreover, our multivariate adaptive regression splines (MARS) study showed that there is a positive correlation in the final IOP when the patients' base IOP is >14 mmHg [18]. Therefore, in this study, we categorized patients into two subgroups based on a base IOP cutoff of 14 mmHg. This article is based on a previous study [18], which identified the key factors influencing end intraocular pressure (IOP) in children receiving atropine treatment. The prior study highlighted the following variables in order of their impact on end IOP: baseline IOP (base IOP), recruitment duration, age, and previous treatment duration, with base IOP being the most significant factor. Additionally, it suggested that atropine may elevate end IOP in children with a baseline IOP greater than 14 mmHg. We incorporated the more prominent influencing factors from the previous analysis as variables (X1–X8) for further examination of their effects on IOP in myopic children undergoing atropine treatment.

We employed ML and SHapley Additive exPlanations (SHAP) to analyze confounders within these IOP subgroups and evaluate their impact on predicting final IOP. This study, to the best of our knowledge, is the first attempt to implement the SHAP module in adolescent patients with myopia treated with atropine. The SHAP module created a personalized and dynamic graphic to illustrate how various factors (e.g., age, sex, cumulative duration, and dosage of atropine treatment) affect the end IOP. This study aimed to predict the end IOP in myopic patients treated with atropine, providing physicians with more individualized insights to enhance patient management and medication safety.

2. Materials and Methods

2.1. Study Design and Protocol

This study, conducted at Shin-Kong Wu Ho-Su Memorial Hospital in Taipei, Taiwan, analyzed data from 2342 eyes of 1171 children diagnosed with myopia and a refractive error of spherical equivalent (SE) less than −10.0D. Data were collected from 1 January 2008 to 31 December 2008, in accordance with the Declaration of Helsinki and approved by the hospital's Institutional Review Board (IRB 20220706R). Exclusions included 324 eyes from participants aged <3 or >18 years; 447 eyes due to loss of follow-up, use of cycloplegics without atropine or presence of ocular diseases including corneal opacity, traumatic injury, uveitis, congenital cataract, congenital glaucoma, optic nerve atrophy, ocular tumor, or prior surgery; and 26 eyes due to use of steroids or anti-glaucoma medications. After exclusions, 1545 eyes from myopic children with regular nightly atropine use remained; 354 eyes were further excluded for irregular drug usage, leaving 1191 individual eyes from 639 boys and 552 girls for analysis. The average age of the whole group was 10.6 ± 2.5 years old. The refractive error of spherical equivalent (SE) in myopia degree was base SE at 2.63D and end SE at 3.12D. The change in myopia degree was −0.48D. Since this article is an extended study based on the order of variables in the previous article, the most important factor affecting end IOP by atropine is base IOP [17]. A previous study suggested that atropine may increase the end IOP in children with a base IOP greater than 14 mmHg [18]. Therefore, base IOP 14 mmHg was used as the basis for grouping, and then the other significant influencing factors in the previous article were further defined as variables (X1–X8) affecting IOP in myopic children undergoing atropine treatment in this article [17,18]. As for the initial myopic degree, since the importance of base SE was less obvious in the previous articles, it was not included in the variable discussion this time. However, atropine is clinically used to treat myopia and is administered according to myopic refraction; children with higher myopia will need more frequent and higher dosages of atropine. Even when myopia occurs earlier, the treatment period will be longer. Therefore, this article currently takes the total cumulative dosage and total medication period into consideration to reflect the relative initial degree of myopia. Patients were divided into two subgroups based on a base IOP cutoff of 14 mmHg, with 619 eyes with a base IOP $\leq$ 14 mmHg and 572 eyes with a base IOP $>$ 14 mmHg. Base IOP was measured using a noncontact tension test (Xpert NCT plus, Reichert, Inc., Depew, NY, USA) and refractive error was assessed using a Canon RK5 autorefractor auto keratometer (Canon Co., Ltd., Tochigi, Japan). The visualization process for preparing the data is shown in Figure 1.

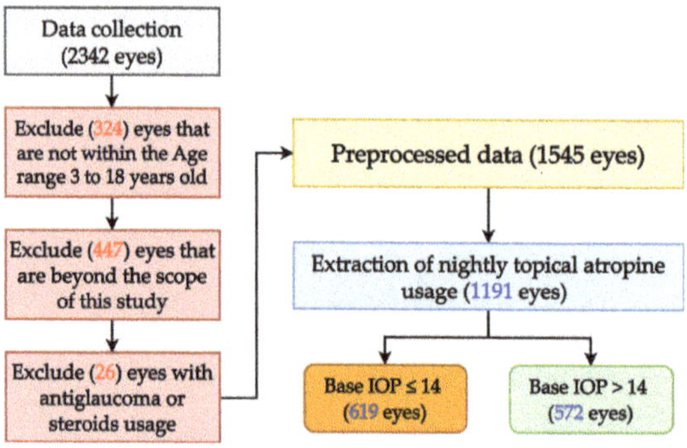

Figure 1. Data preprocessing workflow.

2.2. Variable Definition and Data Description

The study evaluates eight variables (X1–X8) that might affect the end IOP (Y), including sex (X1); age (X2); total follow-up duration (X3); the total cumulative dose of atropine (X4); previous duration (X5); the previous cumulative dose (X6) of atropine use before 1 January 2008; the recruit duration (X7); and the recruit cumulative dose (X8) of atropine use during the study period. This retrospective analysis reviewed patient records from their first visit after 1 January 2005 to their last visit by 30 December 2008, which is represented by X3. Atropine doses were calculated by multiplying the prescribed vial dose (5, 12.5, 25, or 50 mg) by the number of vials and summing these to determine the total cumulative dose (X4). Atropine use after 1 January 2005 but before 1 January 2008 is defined as "previous data", which are also represented by X5 and X6. The recruit atropine treatment was from 1 January 2008 to the last visit on 30 December 2008, which is the period of X7 and X8 being collected. The end IOP (target Y) was recorded as the value from the last visit before the termination of data collection. The descriptive statistics in each subgroup are presented in Table 1.

Table 1. Descriptive statistics of data subgroups.

Variable	Data Subgroups	
	Base IOP ≤ 14	**Base IOP> 14**
	N (%)	
X1: Sex		
1: Male	329 (53%)	310 (54%)
2: Female	290 (47%)	262 (46%)
	Mean (SD)	
X2: Age	10.28 (2.46)	10.96 (2.50)
X3: Total Duration (Months)	19.10 (12.25)	20.31 (12.33)
X4: Total Cumulative Dosage (mg)	116.47 (135.37)	117.62 (137.40)
X5: Previous Duration (Months)	13.54 (12.46)	14.61 (12.37)
X6: Previous Cumulative Dosage (mg)	78.17 (107.27)	77.30 (112.09)
X7: Recruit Duration (Months)	5.53 (3.78)	5.70 (3.72)
X8: Recruit Cumulative Dosage (mg)	38.30 (59.80)	40.32 (63.54)
Y: End IOP (mmHg)	13.83 (2.49)	16.41 (2.44)

2.3. SHapley Additive exPlanations (SHAP)

The interpretability of an ML model may be limited when it comes to explaining individual cases, as ML typically provides a macro/general perspective on the overall data structure. Moreover, the mechanisms could be too complex for clinicians for a straightforward understanding, particularly when trying to discern how specific features influence a target outcome. To address these challenges and improve interpretability, SHAP was utilized in this study. SHAP is a method designed to explain individual predicted outcomes from an ML model by extending the concept of Shapley values from cooperative game theory [19]. SHAP assigns a contribution value to each feature by comparing predictions with and without the feature. This approach considers all possible combinations of features and shows how each feature impacts the predicted outcome, either positively or negatively. Overall, SHAP provides detailed insights into how features influence predictions and has become increasingly popular in clinical studies for explaining feature effects [20,21].

2.4. ML Methods

To examine how features affect end IOP predictions in myopic patients treated with atropine, ML methods were applied for their effectiveness in handling complex feature interactions and common usage in clinical studies [22]. Four ML methods included least absolute shrinkage and selection operator regression (Lasso), classification and regression tree (CART), extreme gradient boosting (XGB), and random forest (RF), which are utilized in this study [23–26]. Each of the utilized ML methods in this study employs distinct strategies to enhance predictive accuracy and feature selection.

Lasso is an extended linear regression method that employs the L1 regularization technique, penalizing the absolute value of coefficients. This penalty encourages sparsity in the model by shrinking less influential coefficients toward zero, effectively selecting only the most impactful features. Lasso's inherent feature selection mechanism makes it particularly effective in reducing overfitting and improving interpretability in high-dimensional datasets.

CART constructs a single regression tree by recursively splitting the data based on variable cutoff points that minimize the prediction error at each step. This approach results in an interpretable decision tree structure, where each split represents a condition on the input variables, ultimately predicting the outcome at the terminal nodes. Furthermore, when constructing the decision tree, the splitting process inherently prioritizes variables that contribute the most to reducing prediction errors, often leaving less relevant features being ignored into the final tree structure.

XGB takes an iterative approach to improving model performance, also known as a boosting approach. By iteratively correcting the residual errors of the previous model under the structure of boosting, XGB enhances accuracy while maintaining computational efficiency. It integrates advanced techniques such as Taylor binomial expansion to speed up convergence, regularization to prevent overfitting, and parallel processing to optimize resource utilization. When constructing XGB, it identifies features that contribute most to reducing the overall error, assigning higher importance to these features through weighted updates. Additionally, XGB includes built-in feature importance metrics, such as gain and cover, to quantify each variable's contribution to the model's performance.

RF is a robust ensemble method that extends the CART approach by building multiple regression trees using randomly selected subsets of the training data and variables. The final prediction from RF is obtained by averaging the predictions from all the individual trees in the forest, reducing variance and improving generalization. This ensemble technique increases robustness and minimizes the likelihood of overfitting compared to a single decision tree. In addition, RF evaluates feature importance based on how much each feature reduces the prediction error across all trees in the forest, with less significant features being ignored or less impactful among the overall RF model.

2.5. Modeling Scheme

Figure 2 illustrates the modeling scheme of this study, which consists of two parts for each base IOP subgroup. The first part involved training the model for 100 rounds to identify the best-performing model; the second part used SHAP to interpret the identified model. As shown in Figure 2, after preparing the base IOP subgroups (as in Figure 1), ML models were repeatedly built. When building models in each round, each ML method required hyper-parameters to be tuned, which is achieved through five-fold cross-validation (5f-CV). 5f-CV randomly divided the training data into five equal folds, with four used for training and one for validation, rotating until all folds were validated. The best hyper-parameter set was chosen based on average validation results, and the model was then tested. Finally, SHAP explained the model with the best testing performance by providing the overall feature rankings and individual case explanations.

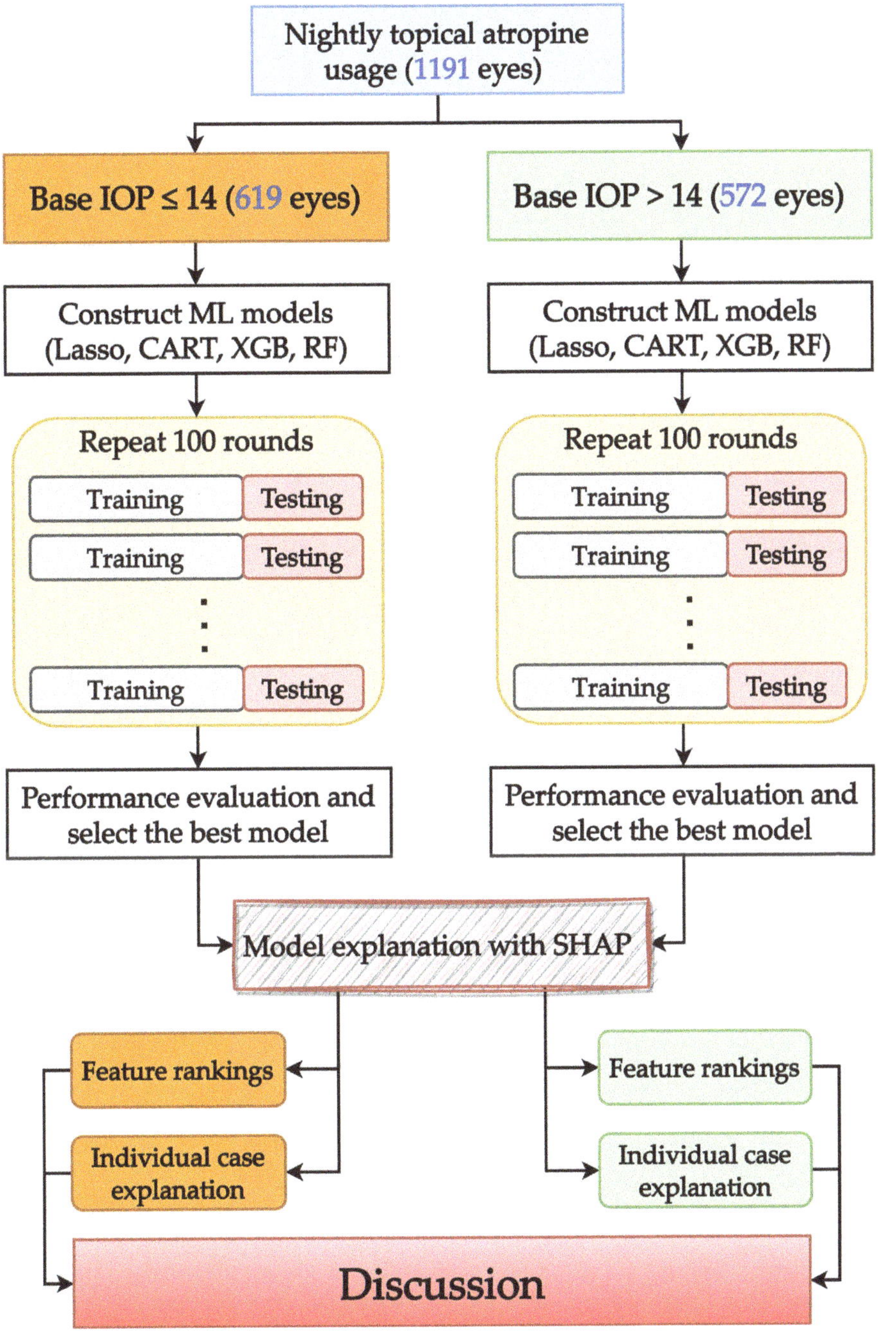

Figure 2. Modeling scheme.

The root mean squared error (RMSE), mean absolute percentage error (MAPE), symmetric mean absolute percentage error (SMAPE), relative absolute error (RAE), and root relative squared error (RRSE) were considered for performance evaluation. Additionally, the experiments in this study were implemented using Python software (version 3.8.8) and related packages.

3. Results

3.1. ML Model Results

To validate the use of ML methods, a multiple linear regression (MLR) model, a standard in clinical studies, was also developed for comparison. Table 2 presents the mean and standard deviation (SD) of 100-round model errors for both base IOP subgroups. In the base IOP $\leq$ 14 subgroup, RF outperformed MLR and all other models across all five error metrics. In the base IOP > 14 subgroup, Lasso performed similarly to MLR, while all the other ML models outperformed MLR. XGB and RF had a comparable MAPE, SMAPE, and RAE, but RF showed the best RMSE (2.37) and RRSE (0.97). Given RF's superior performance in the base IOP $\leq$ 14 subgroup and its better RMSE and RRSE in the base IOP > 14 subgroup, RF was determined to be the best model for further explanation with SHAP.

Table 2. Results of ML models with different subgroup data.

Subgroup	Model	RMSE	MAPE%	SMAPE%	RAE	RRSE
				Mean (SD)		
Base IOP $\leq$ 14	MLR	2.45 (0.16)	14.18 (1.00)	13.64 (0.85)	1.00 (0.02)	1.00 (0.02)
	Lasso	2.44 (0.16)	14.12 (1.00)	13.59 (0.86)	0.99 (0.02)	1.00 (0.01)
	CART	2.47 (0.16)	14.29 (0.98)	13.76 (0.84)	1.01 (0.03)	1.01 (0.03)
	XGB	2.36 (0.15)	13.36 (0.94)	13.02 (0.81)	0.96 (0.05)	0.96 (0.04)
	RF	2.30 (0.15)	13.14 (0.95)	12.74 (0.81)	0.93 (0.05)	0.94 (0.04)
Base IOP > 14	MLR	2.45 (0.20)	12.00 (0.92)	11.69 (0.86)	1.01 (0.02)	1.01 (0.02)
	Lasso	2.45 (0.20)	12.02 (0.91)	11.70 (0.84)	1.01 (0.02)	1.01 (0.01)
	CART	2.43 (0.19)	11.92 (0.91)	11.60 (0.85)	1.00 (0.03)	1.00 (0.03)
	XGB	2.39 (0.19)	11.42 (0.79)	11.27 (0.77)	0.97 (0.04)	0.98 (0.04)
	RF	2.37 (0.19)	11.58 (0.89)	11.30 (0.82)	0.97 (0.05)	0.97 (0.04)

3.2. Feature Importance from SHAP in Each Subgroup

Using SHAP to interpret the best RF model, the overall impact of each feature on end IOP in different base IOP subgroups was visualized, as shown in Figure 3. Panels (a) and (b) correspond to the base IOP $\leq$ 14 subgroup, while panels (c) and (d) correspond to the base IOP > 14 subgroup. Panel (a) shows a SHAP summary plot, where each dot represents the SHAP value for a feature affecting an individual case, with an increasing or decreasing impact on end IOP. The SHAP value of zero serves as a datum point (DP). Dots to the right of DP suggest an increased impact, while those to the left suggest a decreased impact. The color bar on the right displays the actual high/low feature values of an individual case, with higher values appearing in red and lower values in blue.

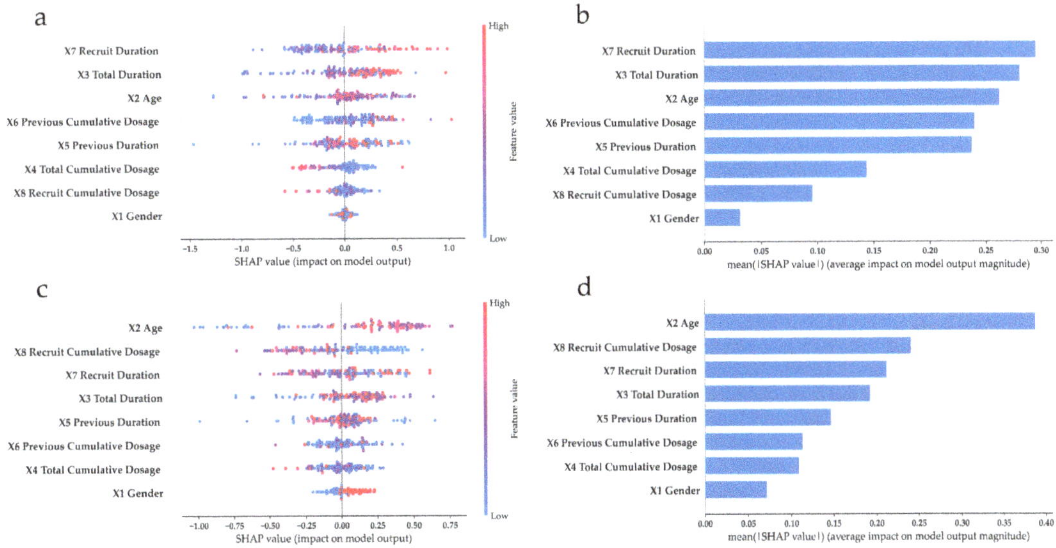

Figure 3. SHAP summary and feature importance plot of each base IOP subgroup. (**a**) SHAP summary plot of base IOP ≤ 14 subgroup. (**b**) SHAP feature importance plot of base IOP ≤ 14 subgroup. (**c**) SHAP summary plot of base IOP > 14 subgroup. (**d**) SHAP feature importance plot of base IOP > 14 subgroup.

The SHAP summary plot provides clinicians an overview of how high/low values of features are likely to affect the end IOP outcome for an individual case. Panel (a) shows that cases with higher values of X7 and X3 are more likely to cause increased end IOP outcomes, as indicated by the concentration of red dots to the right of DP. Moreover, X5 has a mixed influence, varying between cases. To determine the overall impact of a feature, panel (b) averages the absolute SHAP values from panel (a), helping clinicians prioritize the features to be focused. The same concept is followed for panels (c) and (d). In panel (c), it can be found that a lower value of X8 is likely to have increased impact on end IOP, while other medication-related features show mixed effects. Comparing panels (b) and (d), the features have various impacts on the end IOP in different base IOP subgroups. For example, X8 has a greater impact on end IOP in the base IOP > 14 subgroup than in the base IOP ≤ 14 subgroup. Overall, with the aid of SHAP, helpful insights can be generated to learn more about the relationship between atropine use and end IOP.

3.3. *Demonstrations of Individual Case Explanation with SHAP for Each Subgroup*

Understanding how feature values affect end IOP at the individual level is vital for clinicians when planning treatment and determining medication dosages. SHAP aids this process by showing how each feature value influences end IOP outcomes in individual cases using waterfall plots (Figures 4 and 5). Figure 4 presents the example cases in the base IOP ≤ 14 subgroup, while Figure 5 presents the example cases in the base IOP > 14 subgroup.

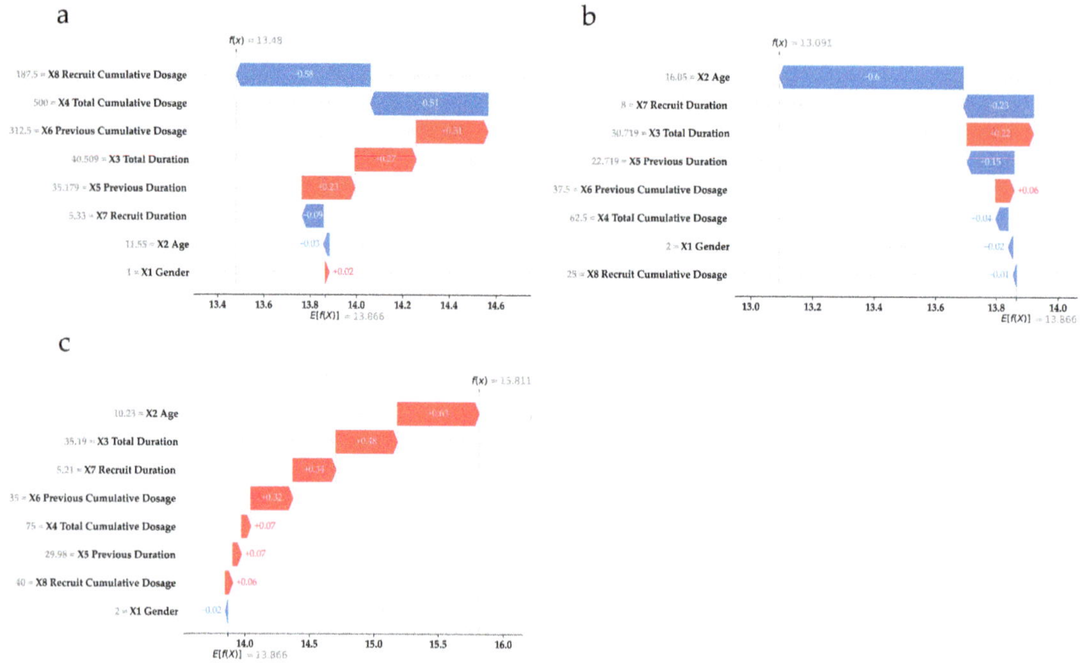

Figure 4. Three examples of individual case (panels (**a**–**c**)) explanations in base IOP $\leq$ 14 subgroup. $f(x)$: model prediction outcome. $E[f(x)]$: expected value.

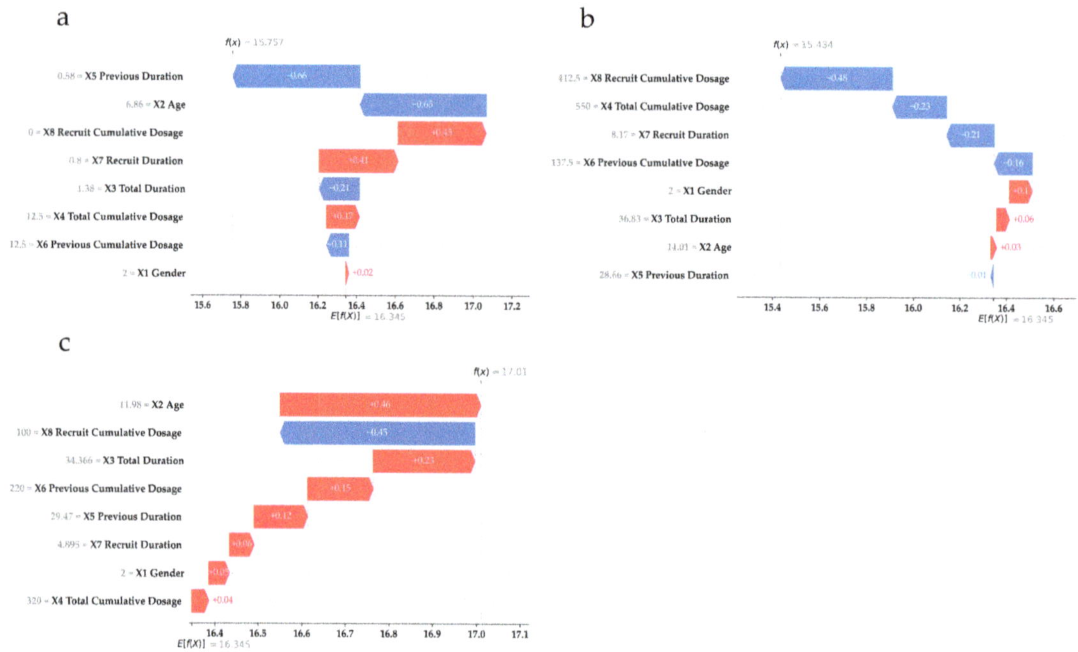

Figure 5. Three examples of individual case (panels (**a**–**c**)) explanations in base IOP > 14 subgroup. $f(x)$: model prediction outcome. $E[f(x)]$: expected value.

Consider panel (a) of Figure 4 as an example for demonstrating how to interpret the waterfall plots. The horizontal axis represents the end IOP value, while the red and blue bars display the increasing and decreasing SHAP values, respectively, representing the contribution of each feature to the final model predicted outcome ($f(x)$, located at the top of the plot). The expected value ($E[f(x)]$, located at the bottom of the plot) is the average end IOP from the data used to train the model, which represents the prediction made without using any features. The final predicted outcome is obtained by adding the expected value and each feature's SHAP value. The vertical axis lists the features and their actual values for each case. Hence, in panel (a), X8 and X4 cause the largest decrease in end IOP for this case.

SHAP helps visualize how feature influences vary between individuals. For example, in panels (e) and (f) of Figure 4, the predicted outcomes are similar (end IOP = 13), but the key features differ. For the case in panel (a), X8 and X4 contributed the most; in panel (b), the largest contributions were from X2 and X7. Moreover, panels (b) and (c) show that even when the same feature (X2) is most influential, impact can vary with different feature values. X2 causes a decreasing impact on end IOP in panel (b) but causes an increasing impact in panel (c).

The same concept applies to Figure 5 for the base IOP > 14 subgroup. For instance, panels (a) and (b) show similar prediction outcomes resulting from different feature contributions. Notably, in panel (c), X2 and X8 offset each other, with X3 being the largest increasing impact contributor. In summary, SHAP illustrates how features and their values influence end IOP outcomes from RF, providing clinicians with detailed insights to better anticipate a patient's potential end IOP with prescribed medications.

4. Discussion

ML models combined with SHAP can rank risk factors and interpret model results [20,21,27]. This study is the first to use ML algorithms with SHAP to analyze confounders across two baseline IOP groups and assess each factor's impact on predicting final IOP in children with myopia treated with atropine. While the average IOP in both groups remained within the normal range, the base IOP was slightly higher in the older group (Table 1) and the end IOP was higher in the base IOP $>$ 14 subgroup. The RF analysis model showed that age (X2) was the most important factor, followed by the cumulative dose (X8) and duration (X7) of atropine (Figure 3, panel [d]). Therefore, older children within base IOP >14 mmHg, their cumulative dosage, and duration of atropine treatment should be closely monitored [28].

The group with a base IOP $\leq$ 14 mmHg is slightly younger, which may contribute to the lower base IOP (Table 1). RF analysis shows that recruit duration (X7) and total duration (X3) are the most important factors influencing end IOP after atropine use (Figure 3, panel [b]). This suggests that even with a lower base IOP in younger patients, a longer history of atropine use could increase the overall treatment duration. Therefore, close monitoring of IOP is essential in long-term atropine therapy, emphasizing the importance of using low-dose atropine to minimize cumulative side effects [7,29].

In panels (b) and (d) of Figure 3, the two groups of children with myopia with different base IOPs, the confounding factors of final IOP, age (X2), and recruit duration (X7) appear among the first three main effects. When using atropine, the longer the medication is taken, the more closely changes in children's IOP need to be monitored. Li et al. [11] conducted a follow-up for the ATOM1 study (atropine 1% vs. placebo; 1999–2003) and the ATOM2 study (atropine 0.01% vs. 0.1% vs. 0.5%; 2006–2012). They compared the 1% atropine-treated group versus the placebo group for the 20-year incidence of cataract/lens opacities, myopic macular degeneration, or parapapillary atrophy (β/γ zone). For children with myopia on long-term atropine, potential sequelae should be monitored and long-term safety tracking is necessary [11].

Our team's previous study, "Identifying and Exploring the Impact Factors for Intraocular Pressure Prediction in Myopic Children with Atropine Control Utilizing Multivariate Adaptive Regression Splines", demonstrated through the MARS model, showed that a baseline intraocular pressure (IOP) exceeding 14 mmHg is associated with an increased risk of elevated end IOP [18]. Building on this finding, the present study provides a more in-depth analysis and extended discussion. In the current study, the average intraocular pressure for the entire cohort changed from an initial 14.5 mmHg to a final 15.07 mmHg, with an average difference of 0.53 mmHg, consistent with our previous findings. Prior biostatistical studies, including both retrospective and prospective analyses, on children with myopia treated with atropine have consistently shown that atropine treatment does not significantly increase the risk of IOP exceeding safety thresholds associated with glaucoma development [16–18].

Given that the significance of baseline spherical equivalent (base SE) was less prominent in earlier studies [17,18], it was not addressed in the current discussion. However, it is well established that the incidence of glaucoma, including normotensive glaucoma, is higher in individuals with myopia [11,28]. Clinically, changes in refraction may influence both treatment regimens and their impact on final intraocular pressure. Future research should focus on a more detailed investigation of refractive changes in relation to myopic progression and their implications for treatment outcomes.

SHAP provided a dynamic RF analysis explanation module, including variables like age, sex, and the duration and dosage of atropine treatment. This study aimed to avoid the risk of a possible increase in IOP when using atropine to treat children with myopia, enabling individualized monitoring of medication safety. In the future, this module could potentially help preset clinical treatment plans based on patient characteristics, whereas the treatment effects can also be monitored as well as the adjustment of therapies if needed. Hence, the module offers clinicians a more precise information policy that would enable more customized and safer treatment. Overall, we hope the SHAP module will help physicians develop more customized and precise atropine treatment plans for myopia control. After treatment, physicians could adjust factors to better meet individual needs, balancing efficacy and safety.

Previously, we used biometric and MARS methods to study the impact of atropine on IOP in children with myopia, finding that the long-term use of atropine alone does not significantly increase IOP [16–18]. However, in recent years, low concentrations of atropine (0.01%) have been combined with corneal reshaping to treat myopia [30]. This combined treatment method has a case report stating that there is a risk of increased IOP [31]. Studies suggest that IOP measurements after removing OK lenses may be falsely lowered due to corneal flattening [32,33]. Therefore, if clinicians encounter atropine and OK lenses combined to treat children with myopia in the future, they must pay more attention to the prediction and tracking of IOP. This article focuses on children with myopia who use atropine alone and reveals the treatment duration and dosage, as well as the patient's personal conditions, such as age, as important variables for the final end IOP. In the future, if myopic treatment becomes more complicated, such as a combination of atropine and OK lenses, more variables can be added to the SHAP module to predict and monitor IOP [5,6,31].

Some limitations of this study need to be addressed. This study's data were hospital-based, with only 1191 eyes analyzed. The predictive accuracy of the SHAP module could further be verified with larger datasets if available. Moreover, atropine is commonly used for treating myopia in children due to the increasing incidence of myopia, which can persist into adolescence. However, the study's treatment duration was only 4 years. Future research should investigate the model's predictive value for IOP over a longer treatment period.

5. Conclusions

This study is the first, to our knowledge, to use the SHAP module to analyze children with myopia treated with topical atropine. SHAP created a personalized graphic illustrating how various factors such as age, sex, and both the previous and cumulative duration and dosage of atropine affect end IOP. In different base IOP subgroups, age (X2) was the most important factor in the base IOP > 14 subgroup, whereas recruit duration (X7) was the one in the base IOP ≤ 14 subgroup. This approach offers clinicians individualized insights to enhance medication safety and patient management.

Author Contributions: Conception and design, project administration: C.-J.L. and T.-E.W.; data collection: J.-W.C., H.-A.C. and T.-E.W.; methods: T.-C.L. and C.-J.L.; writing—original draft preparation: J.-W.C.; analysis and interpretation: J.-W.C., H.-A.C., T.-C.L., T.-E.W. and C.-J.L. All authors have read and agreed to the published version of the manuscript.

Funding: The study was partially supported by the National Science and Technology Council of Taiwan (Grant no. NSTC 112-2221-E-030-011-MY3) and Shin Kong Wu Ho-Su Memorial Hospital (Grant no. 2024SKHADR038).

Institutional Review Board Statement: This research had been performed in accordance with the Declaration of Helsinki and the protocol was approved by the Institutional Review Board of Shin Kong Wu Ho-Su Memorial Hospital (IRB20220706R, Approval date: 8 September 2022). Since this research is retrospective with minimal risk and the potential risks to research subjects are no greater than those for individuals not participating in the research, the exemption from obtaining prior consent does not affect the rights and interests of research subjects.

Informed Consent Statement: The IRB reviewed the research protocol and determined that it is exempt from informed consent.

Data Availability Statement: The datasets generated and/or analyzed during the current study are not publicly available due to privacy/ethical restrictions but are available from the corresponding author upon reasonable request.

Conflicts of Interest: The authors declare that this study was conducted in the absence of any commercial or financial relationships that could be construed as potential conflicts of interest.

References

1. Holden, B.A.; Fricke, T.R.; Wilson, D.A.; Jong, M.; Naidoo, K.S.; Sankaridurg, P.; Wong, T.Y.; Naduvilath, T.J.; Resnikoff, S. Global Prevalence of Myopia and High Myopia and Temporal Trends from 2000 through 2050. *Ophthalmology* **2016**, *123*, 1036–1042. [CrossRef] [PubMed]
2. Sánchez-Tena, M.Á.; Martinez-Perez, C.; Villa-Collar, C.; González-Pérez, M.; González-Abad, A.; Grupo de Investigación Alain Afflelou; Alvarez-Peregrina, C. Prevalence and Estimation of the Evolution of Myopia in Spanish Children. *J. Clin. Med.* **2024**, *13*, 1800. [CrossRef] [PubMed]
3. Eppenberger, L.S.; Jaggi, G.P.; Todorova, M.G.; Messerli, J.; Sturm, V. Following prevalence of myopia in a large Swiss military cohort over the last decade: Where is the European "myopia boom"? *Graefe's Arch. Clin. Exp. Ophthalmol.* **2024**, *262*, 3039–3046. [CrossRef] [PubMed]
4. Mutti, D.O.; Sinnott, L.T.; Cotter, S.A.; Jones-Jordan, L.A.; Kleinstein, R.N.; Manny, R.E.; Twelker, J.D.; Zadnik, K. Predicting the onset of myopia in children by age, sex, and ethnicity: Results from the CLEERE Study. *Optom. Vis. Sci. Off. Publ. Am. Acad. Optom.* **2024**, *101*, 179–186. [CrossRef]
5. Du, L.F.; He, F.; Tan, H.X.; Gao, N.; Song, W.Q.; Luo, Y.X. Comparisons of Three Methods for Myopia Control in Adolescents. *J. Ophthalmol.* **2022**, *2022*, 9920002. [CrossRef]
6. Wang, Z.; Wang, P.; Jiang, B.; Meng, Y.; Qie, S.; Yan, Z. The efficacy and safety of 0.01% atropine alone or combined with orthokeratology for children with myopia: A meta-analysis. *PLoS ONE* **2023**, *18*, e0282286. [CrossRef]

7. Yam, J.C.; Zhang, X.J.; Zhang, Y.; Yip, B.H.K.; Tang, F.; Wong, E.S.; Bui, C.H.T.; Kam, K.W.; Ng, M.P.H.; Ko, S.T.; et al. Effect of Low-Concentration Atropine Eyedrops vs Placebo on Myopia Incidence in Children: The LAMP2 Randomized Clinical Trial. *JAMA* **2023**, *329*, 472–481. [CrossRef]
8. Chia, A.; Ngo, C.; Choudry, N.; Yamakawa, Y.; Tan, D. Atropine Ophthalmic Solution to Reduce Myopia Progression in Pediatric Subjects: The Randomized, Double-Blind Multicenter Phase II APPLE Study. *Asia-Pac. J. Ophthalmol.* **2023**, *12*, 370–376. [CrossRef]
9. Kuo, H.Y.; Ke, C.H.; Chen, S.T.; Sun, H.Y. The Impact of Clinical Atropine Use in Taiwanese Schoolchildren: Changes in Physiological Characteristics and Visual Functions. *Children* **2021**, *8*, 1054. [CrossRef]
10. Cyphers, B.; Huang, J.; Walline, J.J. Symptoms and ocular findings associated with administration of 0.01% atropine in young adults. *Clin. Exp. Optom.* **2023**, *106*, 311–321. [CrossRef]
11. Li, Y.; Yip, M.; Ning, Y.; Chung, J.; Toh, A.; Leow, C.; Liu, N.; Ting, D.; Schmetterer, L.; Saw, S.M.; et al. Topical Atropine for Childhood Myopia Control: The Atropine Treatment Long-Term Assessment Study. *JAMA Ophthalmol.* **2024**, *142*, 15–23. [CrossRef] [PubMed]
12. Wang, M.; Cui, C.; Yu, S.A.; Liang, L.L.; Ma, J.X.; Fu, A.C. Effect of 0.02% and 0.01% atropine on ocular biometrics: A two-year clinical trial. *Front. Pediatr.* **2023**, *11*, 1095495. [CrossRef] [PubMed]
13. Rengstorff, R.H.; Doughty, C.B. Mydriatic and cycloplegic drugs: A review of ocular and systemic complications. *Am. J. Optom. Physiol. Opt.* **1982**, *59*, 162–177. [CrossRef] [PubMed]
14. Guier, C.P. Elevated intraocular pressure and myopic shift linked to topiramate use. *Optom. Vis. Sci. Off. Publ. Am. Acad. Optom.* **2007**, *84*, 1070–1073. [CrossRef]
15. Sihota, R.; Tuli, D.; Dada, T.; Gupta, V.; Sachdeva, M.M. Distribution and determinants of intraocular pressure in a normal pediatric population. *J. Pediatr. Ophthalmol. Strabismus* **2006**, *43*, 14–37. [CrossRef]
16. Yu, T.C.; Wu, T.E.; Wang, Y.S.; Cheng, S.F.; Liou, S.W. A STROBE-compliant case-control study: Effects of cumulative doses of topical atropine on intraocular pressure and myopia progression. *Medicine* **2020**, *99*, e22745. [CrossRef]
17. Wu, T.E.; Chen, H.A.; Jhou, M.J.; Chen, Y.N.; Chang, T.J.; Lu, C.J. Evaluating the Effect of Topical Atropine Use for Myopia Control on Intraocular Pressure by Using Machine Learning. *J. Clin. Med.* **2020**, *10*, 111. [CrossRef]
18. Wu, T.E.; Chen, J.W.; Liu, T.C.; Yu, C.H.; Jhou, M.J.; Lu, C.J. Identifying and Exploring the Impact Factors for Intraocular Pressure Prediction in Myopic Children with Atropine Control Utilizing Multivariate Adaptive Regression Splines. *J. Pers. Med.* **2024**, *14*, 125. [CrossRef]
19. Lundberg, S.M.; Lee, S.I. A Unified Approach to Interpreting Model Predictions. In Proceedings of the 31st International Conference on Neural Information Processing Systems, Long Beach, CA, USA, 4–9 December 2017; pp. 4768–4777.
20. Sun, J.; Sun, C.K.; Tang, Y.X.; Liu, T.C.; Lu, C.J. Application of SHAP for Explainable Machine Learning on Age-Based Subgrouping Mammography Questionnaire Data for Positive Mammography Prediction and Risk Factor Identification. *Healthcare* **2023**, *11*, 2000. [CrossRef]
21. Li, J.; Dai, Y.; Mu, Z.; Wang, Z.; Meng, J.; Meng, T.; Wang, J. Choice of refractive surgery types for myopia assisted by machine learning based on doctors' surgical selection data. *BMC Med. Inform. Decis. Mak.* **2024**, *24*, 41. [CrossRef]
22. Breeze, F.; Hossain, R.R.; Mayo, M.; McKelvie, J. Predicting ophthalmic clinic non-attendance using machine learning: Development and validation of models using nationwide data. *Clin. Exp. Ophthalmol.* **2023**, *51*, 764–774. [CrossRef] [PubMed]
23. Tibshirani, R. Regression shrinkage and selection via the lasso. *J. R. Stat. Soc. Ser. B Stat. Methodol.* **1996**, *58*, 267–288. [CrossRef]
24. Breiman, L.; Friedman, J.H.; Olshen, R.A.; Stone, C.J. *Classification and Regression Trees*, 1st ed.; Routledge: Abingdon, UK, 1984.
25. Chen, T.; Guestrin, C. XGBoost: A Scalable Tree Boosting System. In Proceedings of the 22nd ACM SIGKDD International Conference on Knowledge Discovery and Data Mining, San Francisco, CA, USA, 13–17 August 2016; pp. 785–794.
26. Ho, T.K. Random decision forests. In Proceedings of the 3rd International Conference on Document Analysis and Recognition, Montreal, QC, Canada, 14–16 August 1995; pp. 278–282.
27. Tsay, S.F.; Chang, C.Y.; Shueh Hung, S.; Su, J.Y.; Kuo, C.Y.; Mu, P.F. Pain prediction model based on machine learning and SHAP values for elders with dementia in Taiwan. *Int. J. Med. Inform.* **2024**, *188*, 105475. [CrossRef]
28. Lee, E.J.; Lee, D.; Kim, M.J.; Kim, K.; Han, J.C.; Kee, C. Different glaucoma progression rates by age groups in young myopic glaucoma patients. *Sci Rep.* **2024**, *14*, 2589. [CrossRef] [PubMed] [PubMed Central]
29. Tsuda, H.; Someko, H.; Kataoka, Y. Low-Concentration Atropine Eyedrops for Myopia in Children. *JAMA* **2023**, *329*, 1885–1886. [CrossRef]
30. Zheng, N.N.; Tan, K.W. The synergistic efficacy and safety of combined low-concentration atropine and orthokeratology for slowing the progression of myopia: A meta-analysis. *Ophthalmic Physiol. Opt. J. Br. Coll. Ophthalmic Opt.* **2022**, *42*, 1214–1226. [CrossRef]

31. Lee, Y.R.; Hwang, J.; Kim, J.S. Increase of Intraocular Pressure after Application of 0. *125% Atropine Eye Drops in Children Using Ortho-K Contact Lenses. Case Rep. Ophthalmol.* **2024**, *15*, 292–297. [CrossRef]
32. Chang, C.J.; Yang, H.H.; Chang, C.A.; Wu, R.; Tsai, H.Y. The influence of orthokeratology on intraocular pressure measurements. *Semin. Ophthalmol.* **2013**, *28*, 210–215. [CrossRef]
33. Ishida, Y.; Yanai, R.; Sagara, T.; Nishida, T.; Toshida, H.; Murakami, A. Decrease in intraocular pressure following orthokeratology measured with a noncontact tonometer. *Jpn. J. Ophthalmol.* **2011**, *55*, 190–195. [CrossRef]

medicina

MDPI

Article

Changes in Protein Expression in Warmed Human Lens Epithelium Cells Using Shotgun Proteomics

Hiroko Otake [1,†], Tetsushi Yamamoto [1,†], Naoki Yamamoto [2], Yosuke Nakazawa [3], Yoshiki Miyata [4], Atsushi Taga [1], Hiroshi Sasaki [5] and Noriaki Nagai [1,*]

1 Faculty of Pharmacy, Kindai University, Osaka 577-8502, Japan
2 Research Promotion Headquarters, Fujita Health University, Toyoake 470-1192, Japan
3 Faculty of Pharmacy, Keio University, 1-5-30 Shibakoen, Tokyo 105-8512, Japan
4 Faculty of Pharmacy, Teikyo University, 2-11-1 Kaga, Tokyo 173-8606, Japan
5 Department of Ophthalmology, Kanazawa Medical University, Uchinada 920-0293, Japan
* Correspondence: nagai_n@phar.kindai.ac.jp; Tel.: +81-6-4307-3638
† These authors contributed equally to this work.

Abstract: *Background and Objectives*: In previous studies, we reported that the assessment of the cumulative thermal dose in the crystalline lens, conducted through computational modeling utilizing a supercomputer and the biothermal transport equation, exhibited a significant association with the incidence of nuclear cataracts. In this study, we have investigated the types of proteins that expressed underlying 35.0 °C (normal-temp) and 37.5 °C (warming-temp) by using the shotgun liquid chromatography (LC) with tandem mass spectrometry (MS/MS)-based global proteomic approach. *Materials and Methods*: We have discussed the changes in protein expression in warmed iHLEC-NY2 cells using Gene Ontology analysis and a label-free semiquantitative method based on spectral counting. *Results*: In iHLEC-NY2, 615 proteins were detected, including 307 (49.9%) present in both lenses cultured at normal-temp and warming-temp, 130 (21.1%) unique to the lens cultured at normal-temp, and 178 (29.0%) unique to the lens cultured at warming-temp. Furthermore, LC–MS/MS analysis showed that warming decreased the expression of actin, alpha cardiac muscle 1, actin-related protein 2, putative tubulin-like protein alpha-4B, ubiquitin carboxyl-terminal hydrolase 17-like protein 1, ubiquitin-ribosomal protein eL40 fusion protein, ribosome biogenesis protein BMS1 homolog, histone H2B type 1-M, and histone H2A.J. in iHLEC-NY2. *Conclusions*: The decreases in the specific protein levels of actin, tubulin, ubiquitin, ribosomes, and histones may be related to cataract development under warming conditions. This investigation could provide a critical framework for understanding the correlation between temperature dynamics and the development of nuclear cataracts.

Keywords: shotgun proteomics; lens; temperature; cataract; iHLEC-NY2

1. Introduction

Cataracts are a leading cause of blindness worldwide. With the increasing lifespan worldwide, the number of individuals whose sight is threatened by this disease is expected to increase. There are four major types of cataracts: cortical, nuclear, posterior subcapsular, and mixed. Different risk factors were associated with each risk type. Epidemiological research has identified multiple factors that are linked to an elevated risk of developing nuclear cataracts (NUCs), including greater sunlight exposure, lower socioeconomic status, poorer nutrition, smoking, cortical cataracts due to diabetes, greater sunlight exposure, and female sex [1–4]. NUCs have the greatest clinical significance because they are the most common type of cataracts and occur along the visual axis. Treatments that prevent the appearance or delay the progression of NUCs have significant therapeutic value. Previous research has shown that the prevalence of NUCs, graded at level ≥ 1 according to the World Health Organization (WHO) cataract grading system, was notably higher in tropical and subtropical regions than in temperate and subarctic regions, regardless of racial factors [5–7]. Therefore, elevated lens temperatures resulting from higher environmental temperatures may contribute to an increased risk of NUC formation.

Thus, we hypothesized that the occurrence of cataracts is associated with environmental temperature. The supporting evidence includes a study on ambient temperature effects, where the lens temperature of monkeys exposed to direct sunlight at 49 °C increased to 41 °C within 10 min [8]. Similarly, in rabbits, the lens temperature decreased by 7 °C when maintained in an environment at 4 °C [9]. Another rabbit-based experiment demonstrated significant correlations between ambient temperature under sunlight and the temperatures of the lens and posterior chamber aqueous humor [8].

In this study, we investigated the relationship between environmental temperature and lens temperature through an in silico computer simulation. The lens temperature was estimated to range between 35 °C and 37.5 °C depending on the ambient temperature surrounding the eyeball. However, when the ambient temperature exceeded 30 °C, the estimated lens temperature varied with age, showing an increase in older individuals [10]. Our study showed that, as environmental temperatures rise, the temperature of the eye lens increases to 35–37.5 °C or higher, which correlates with the development of NUCs. The temperature increase, particularly in the lens nucleus, coincides with the opacity area of the cataract. When the lens temperature exceeds 37.5 °C, cumulative heat exposure is positively correlated with NUC incidence [5,10]. This suggests that prolonged exposure to elevated temperatures, especially with aging, may increase the risk of developing NUCs. In addition, we previously investigated the relationship between temperature and NUC incidence in the rat whole lens (including the epithelium, cortex, and nucleus) using a shotgun proteomic analysis approach and showed that the levels of actin, tubulin, vimentin, filensin, and fatty acid-binding protein 5 decreased under warming-temperatures (37.5 °C) [11]. However, it remains unclear whether similar results can be obtained in the human lens, and the detailed mechanisms underlying these findings have yet to be elucidated.

Based on this background, identifying the expression of proteins that fluctuate under warming conditions in human lens cells and discussing preventive measures could contribute to the clinical prevention of NUCs. In this study, we employed a shotgun proteomic analysis approach [12,13] in iHLEC-NY2 (human lens epithelial cells) to investigate the cataractous factors that are relevant to normal and warming conditions.

2. Materials and Methods

2.1. Culture Cells

The immortalized human lens epithelial cell line iHLEC-NY2 was used as described by Yamamoto et al. [14]. Briefly, the iHLEC-NY2 cell line (source of the cell line "Fujita Health University, Research Promotion Headquarters"), derived from human lens epithelial cells and transfected with modified SV40 large T antigen [15,16], was cultured in medium containing FBS, bFGF, GlutaMAXTM I, DMEM/F12, and penicillin–streptomycin. Cells were cultured at 35.0 °C (normal-temp) and 37.5 °C (warming-temp) in a 5% CO_2 incubator. The experiment using iHLEC-NY2 was approved by the Ethic Review Committee of Fujita Health University (No. 004, approval date 1 April 2021) and Kanazawa Medical University

Biosafety Committee for Recombinant DNA Research (Approval No. 2020-18, approval date 11 November 2020).

2.2. *Tryptic Digestion of Proteins Extracted from iHLEC-NY2*

iHLEC-NY2 cells were homogenized using at the Minute™ total protein extraction kit for mass spectrometry (Invent Biotechnologies, Inc., Plymouth, MN, USA). Protein concentrations were determined using the Bio-Rad Protein Assay Kit (Bio-Rad Laboratories, Inc., Hercules, CA, USA). Gel-free trypsin digestion was performed as previously described [17]. Briefly, 10 μg of protein extract from each sample was reduced at 37.5 °C for 30 min using 20 mM Tris(2-carboxyethyl)phosphine in 50 mM ammonium bicarbonate buffer and 45 mM dithiothreitol. Subsequently, the proteins were alkylated with 100 mM iodoacetamide in 50 mM ammonium bicarbonate buffer at 37.5 °C for 30 min. Following this alkylation, the samples were digested at 37.5 °C for 24 h using MS-grade trypsin gold (Promega Corp., Madison, WI, USA) at a trypsin-to-protein ratio of 1:100 (*w*:*w*). Finally, the digested peptides were purified using PepClean C-18 Spin Columns (Thermo Fisher Scientific, Waltham, MA, USA) according to the manufacturer's instructions.

2.3. *Identification of Proteins*

The analysis was performed following our previous study [12,13]. Briefly, peptide samples (2 μg) were injected using a peptide L-trap column (Chemicals Evaluation and Research Institute, Tokyo, Japan) and HTC PAL autosampler (CTC Analytics, Zwingen, Switzerland). Peptide separation occurred on a Paradigm MS4 system (AMR Inc., Tokyo, Japan) with a reverse-phase C18 column (L-column, 3-μm gel particles, 120 Å pore size, and 0.2 mm × 150 mm) at a flow rate of 1 μL/min. The mobile phase consisted of 0.1% formic acid in water (solution A) and acetonitrile (solution B), with gradient elution from 5% to 40% solution B over 120 min. Peptides were analyzed using an LTQ ion-trap mass spectrometer (Thermo Fisher Scientific, Inc.) without sheath or auxiliary gas. MS scan sequences included full-scan MS followed by MS/MS of the two most intense peaks, with parameters optimized for fragmentation. MS/MS data were searched against the SwissProt database using Mascot version 2.4.01, enabling trypsin digestion, missed cleavages, and modifications such as cysteine carbamidomethylation and methionine oxidation. In this study, the fold change in expression was determined as the log2-transformed ratio of protein abundance (*Rsc*) and assessed via spectral counting [18]. *Rsc* was calculated by Equation (1) as follows:

$$Rsc = log_2\frac{n_s + f}{n_n + f} + log_2\frac{t_n + n_n + f}{t_s + n_s - f} \quad (1)$$

In addition, the normalized spectral abundance factor (*NSAF*) [19] was computed by Equation (2) as follows:

$$NSAF = \frac{SpC_n/L_n}{SUM(SpC_n/L_n)} \quad (2)$$

Here, n_n and n_s represent the spectral counts for proteins in rat retinas, whereas t_n and t_s indicate the total spectral counts for all proteins in each sample. The correction factor, denoted as f, was 1.25. SpC_n refers to the spectral count of the protein in rat lenses incubated at normal-temp and warming-temp, while L_n denotes the protein length in these conditions. Proteins were considered differentially expressed when the *Rsc* value was greater than 2 or less than −2, which corresponded to fold changes greater than 2 or less than 0.5, respectively.

2.4. Bioinformatics

This study explored the roles of proteins that exhibited notable changes under normal and warming conditions. The sequences were annotated by assigning Gene Ontology (GO) terms corresponding to molecular functions, cellular components, and biological processes, along with Kyoto Encyclopedia of Genes and Genomes (KEGG) signaling pathways, utilizing the Database for Annotation, Visualization, and Integrated Discovery (DAVID, https://davidbioinformatics.nih.gov/tools.jsp, accessed on 3 February 2025) [20–22]. Additionally, p-values for the GO analysis were computed through this database tool.

3. Results

Protein Expression in iHLEC-NY2 With or Without Warming

Amounts of 437 and 485 proteins were identified in iHLEC-NY2 cultured at normal-temp and warming-temp, respectively (Figure 1A). Moreover, 615 proteins were detected in iHLEC-NY2, including 307 (49.9%) present in both lenses cultured at normal-temp and warming-temp, 130 (21.1%) unique to the lens cultured at normal-temp, and 178 (29.0%) unique to the lens cultured at warming-temp (Figure 1A). Next, we investigated the proteins expressed in the iHLEC-NY2 cells. Figure 1B shows the Rsc values for the proteins identified in the lenses cultured at normal-temp and warming-temp. A positive Rsc value indicated enhanced expression of proteins in the iHLEC-NY2 cells cultured at elevated temperatures, while a negative value signified reduced expression. Additionally, the NSAF value was computed for each protein identified in iHLEC-NY2 cells cultured at both normal- and warming-temp. Proteins with Rsc values greater than 2 or less than −2 were identified as candidate proteins exhibiting differential regulation in response to the different culture conditions. At different culture temperatures, the housekeeping protein levels (GAPDH, glyceraldehyde-3-phosphate dehydrogenase) did not change.

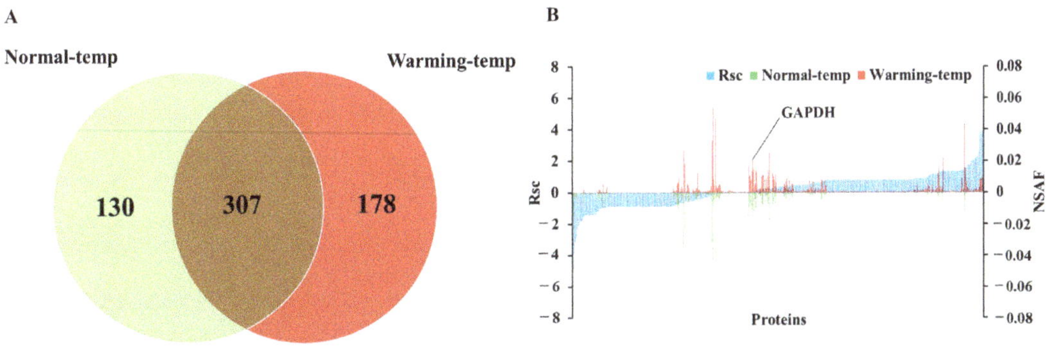

Figure 1. Identification and semiquantitative comparison of the differentially expressed proteins in iHLEC-NY2 cells cultured at normal-temp and warming-temp. (**A**) Venn diagram depicting proteins identified in iHLEC-NY2 cells grown at normal-temp and warming-temp. (**B**) Semiquantitative analysis of proteins differentially expressed in iHLEC-NY2 cells cultured at warming-temp. To compare the expression levels of identified proteins between cells cultured at normal-temp and warming-temp, Rsc and NSAF values were calculated. The blue peak represents Rsc, while the green and red peaks correspond to the NSAF values at normal-temp (lower peak) and warming-temp (upper peak), respectively. Rsc is plotted such that its expression increases from left to right under warming-temp, providing a visual representation of the detected protein behavior. When focusing on GAPDH as a housekeeping protein, it is detected at the approximate center of the x-axis, with NSAF values at normal- (lower peak) and warming-temp (upper peak) showing similar intensities. This consistency suggests that the semiquantitative analysis of proteins was conducted appropriately.

We performed a GO analysis on the candidate proteins regulated in the iHLEC-NY2 cells cultured at elevated temperatures. For this analysis, we queried GO terms using the DAVID database, and the results of "molecular function", "cellular component", "biological processes", and "KEGG pathway" are shown in Tables 1–4, respectively. In the categories of "molecular function", "cellular component", "biological processes", and "KEGG pathway", the detected counts were 29, 44, 43, and 16, respectively. Among these, the most abundant terms in each category were "protein binding", "extracellular exosome", "nucleosome assembly", and "neutrophil extracellular trap formation", respectively.

Table 1. GO analysis of identified proteins in molecular function category.

Molecular Function Category	Relative Abundance (%)	Molecular Function Category	Relative Abundance (%)
Protein binding	77.1	Unfolded protein binding	6.37
RNA binding	32.5	Structural molecule activity	5.73
DNA binding	29.3	Structural constituent of muscle	4.46
Protein heterodimerization activity	28.0	Double-stranded DNA binding	3.18
Structural constituent of chromatin	27.4	Protein binding involved in protein folding	3.18
ATP binding	15.9	Collagen binding	2.55
Protein domain specific binding	12.1	Heat shock protein binding	2.55
Cadherin binding	11.5	Microfilament motor activity	2.55
GTP binding	8.28	Misfolded protein binding	2.55
Structural constituent of cytoskeleton	8.28	Motor activity	2.55
ATPase activity	7.64	Structural constituent of epidermis	2.55
GTPase activity	7.64	mRNA 5′-UTR binding	1.91
Structural constituent of ribosome	7.64	Protein disulfide isomerase activity	1.91
Actin binding	6.37	Large ribosomal subunit rRNA binding	1.27
Actin filament binding	6.37		

Table 2. GO analysis of identified proteins in cellular component category.

Cellular Component Category	Relative Abundance (%)	Cellular Component Category	Relative Abundance (%)
Extracellular exosome	63.7	Cytosolic large ribosomal subunit	4.46
Nucleus	58.6	Ribonucleoprotein complex	4.46
Cytosol	53.5	Cytosolic small ribosomal subunit	3.82
Cytoplasm	41.4	Ficolin-1-rich granule lumen	3.82
Nucleoplasm	39.5	Actin filament	3.18
Membrane	36.9	Meiotic spindle	3.18
Nucleosome	28.0	Small-subunit processome	3.18
Extracellular region	22.9	Vesicle	3.18
Macromolecular complex	21.7	Z disc	3.18
Focal adhesion	15.3	Intercellular bridge	2.55
Nuclear chromosome	15.3	Myosin complex	2.55
Extracellular space	14.7	Myosin II complex	2.55
Endoplasmic reticulum	12.7	Ruffle membrane	2.55
CENP-A-containing nucleosome	10.2	Sarcomere	2.55
Chromosome, telomeric region	10.2	Small ribosomal subunit	2.55
Perinuclear region of cytoplasm	8.28	Smooth endoplasmic reticulum	2.55
Ribosome	8.28	Endoplasmic reticulum chaperone complex	1.91
Cytosolic ribosome	7.01	Myosin filament	1.91
Melanosome	5.73	Polysome	1.91
Endoplasmic reticulum lumen	5.10	CRD-mediated mRNA stability complex	1.27
Intermediate filament	5.10	Muscle thin filament tropomyosin	1.27
Microtubule	5.10	Myosin II filament	1.27

Table 3. GO analysis of identified proteins in biological process category.

Cellular Component Category	Relative Abundance (%)	Cellular Component Category	Relative Abundance (%)
Nucleosome assembly	23.6	Cytoskeleton organization	3.82
Chromatin organization	17.2	Microtubule-based process	3.82
DNA replication-dependent nucleosome assembly	15.3	Actomyosin structure organization	3.18
Telomere organization	15.3	Muscle contraction	3.18
Protein localization to CENP-A containing chromatin	10.2	Oocyte maturation	3.18
DNA-templated transcription, initiation	9.55	Osteoblast differentiation	3.18
DNA replication-independent nucleosome assembly	8.92	Ribosomal small subunit biogenesis	3.18
Negative regulation of megakaryocyte differentiation	8.92	Spindle assembly involved in female meiosis	3.18
Cytoplasmic translation	7.64	Cellular response to unfolded protein	2.55
Negative regulation of apoptotic process	7.64	Chaperone mediated protein folding requiring cofactor	2.55
Translation	7.64	Protein folding in endoplasmic reticulum	2.55
Gene expression	7.01	Protein refolding	2.55
Regulation of gene expression, epigenetic	6.37	Actin filament-based movement	2.55
Protein folding	5.73	Cellular copper ion homeostasis	1.91
Antibacterial humoral response	5.10	Cellular response to interleukin-7	1.91
Antimicrobial humoral immune response mediated by antimicrobial peptide	5.10	Dendritic spine organization	1.91
Defense response to Gram-positive bacterium	5.10	Long-term synaptic depression	1.91
Heterochromatin assembly	5.10	Mitotic cleavage furrow ingression	1.91
Innate immune response in mucosa	5.10	Regulation of Arp2/3 complex-mediated actin nucleation	1.91
Mitotic cell cycle	5.10	Regulation of receptor internalization	1.91
Intermediate filament organization	4.46	Skeletal muscle myosin thick filament assembly	1.27
Microtubule cytoskeleton organization	4.46		

Table 4. GO analysis of identified proteins in pathway category.

Molecular Function Category	Relative Abundance (%)	Molecular Function Category	Relative Abundance (%)
Neutrophil extracellular trap formation	26.7	Protein processing in endoplasmic reticulum	6.37
Alcoholism	25.5	Motor proteins	5.73
Systemic lupus erythematosus	25.5	Parkinson disease	5.73
Viral carcinogenesis	17.2	Prion disease	5.73
Shigellosis	9.55	Pathogenic Escherichia coli infection	5.10
Coronavirus disease—COVID-19	7.01	Necroptosis	4.46
Ribosome	7.01	Estrogen signaling pathway	3.82
Transcriptional misregulation in cancer	7.01	Antigen processing and presentation	3.18

In addition, we listed proteins with expression changes at warming-temp that showed Rsc > 2 or <−2 via the label-free semiquantitative method based on spectral counting (Tables 5 and 6). The proteins demonstrating Rsc > 2 or <−2 were detected to be 30 in total, and, at warming-temp, the expression levels of 19 proteins were upregulated, while the expression levels of another 11 proteins were downregulated. In this study, our focus was on the downregulated proteins at warming-temp since they are more prone to being influenced than overexpressed proteins. The factors in this study were actin, alpha cardiac muscle 1, actin-related protein 2, putative tubulin-like protein alpha-4B, ubiquitin carboxyl-terminal hydrolase 17-like protein 1, ubiquitin-ribosomal protein eL40 fusion protein, ribosome biogenesis protein BMS1 homolog, histone H2B type 1-M, and histone H2A.J. Keratin was also detected via proteomic analysis. However, because keratin is not present in the lens, the possibility of contamination during lens extraction has been suggested.

Table 5. Semiquantitative comparison of proteins with increased expression in iHLEC-NY2 cultured under warming-temp conditions.

ID	Accession Number and Description		Number of Amino Acids	Spectral Counting		
				Warming-Temp	Normal-Temp	Fold Change, Rsc
TBA1C_HUMAN	Q9BQE3	Tubulin alpha-1C chain	449	89	0	6.156903
HS902_HUMAN	Q14568	Heat shock protein HSP 90-alpha	343	21	0	4.122102
H2B1C_HUMAN	P62807	Histone H2B type 1-C/E/F/G/I	126	18	0	3.912511
H2BFS_HUMAN	P57053	Histone H2B type F-S	126	17	0	3.834335
H2B1D_HUMAN	P58876	Histone H2B type 1-D	126	17	0	3.834335
H2A1H_HUMAN	Q96KK5	Histone H2A type 1-H	128	16	0	3.753820
H31_HUMAN	P68431	Histone H3.1	136	7	0	2.687759
RS3A_HUMAN	P61247	Small ribosomal subunit protein eS1	264	6	0	2.501132
PGAM2_HUMAN	P15259	Phosphoglycerate mutase 2	253	5	0	2.286793
RLA0L_HUMAN	Q8NHW5	Putative ribosomal protein uL10-like	317	5	0	2.286793
TGM2_HUMAN	P21980	Protein-glutamine gamma-glutamyltransferase 2	687	19	3	2.219596
HS71L_HUMAN	P34931	Heat shock 70 kDa protein 1-like	641	14	2	2.196653
HSP76_HUMAN	P17066	Heat shock 70 kDa protein 6	643	18	3	2.146318
CNGB1_HUMAN	Q14028	Cyclic nucleotide-gated cation channel beta-1	1251	4	0	2.035040
RPN1_HUMAN	P04843	Dolichyl-diphosphooligosaccharide--protein glycosyltransferase subunit 1	607	4	0	2.035040
RL15_HUMAN	P61313	Large ribosomal subunit protein eL15	204	4	0	2.035040
MYH14_HUMAN	Q7Z406	Myosin-14	1995	4	0	2.035040
TAF9B_HUMAN	Q9HBM6	Transcription initiation factor TFIID subunit 9B	251	4	0	2.035040
PDIA4_HUMAN	P13667	Protein disulfide-isomerase A4	645	8	1	2.004817

Table 6. Semiquantitative comparison of proteins with decreased expression in iHLEC-NY2 cultured under warming-temp conditions.

ID	Accession Number and Description		Number of Amino Acids	Spectral Counting		
				Warming-Temp	Normal-Temp	Fold Change, Rsc
ACTC_HUMAN	P68032	Actin, alpha cardiac muscle 1	377	0	81	6.094116
H2B1M_HUMAN	Q99879	Histone H2B type 1-M	126	0	34	4.861313
K2C75_HUMAN	O95678	Keratin, type II cytoskeletal 75	551	0	16	3.826320
H2AJ_HUMAN	Q9BTM1	Histone H2A.J	129	0	10	3.208328
TBA4B_HUMAN	Q9H853	Putative tubulin-like protein alpha-4B	241	0	9	3.073807
K1C26_HUMAN	Q7Z3Y9	Keratin, type I cytoskeletal 26	468	0	8	2.925489
U17L1_HUMAN	Q7RTZ2	Ubiquitin carboxyl-terminal hydrolase 17-like protein 1	530	0	7	2.760210
K2C79_HUMAN	Q5XKE5	Keratin, type II cytoskeletal 79	535	0	5	2.359232
RL40_HUMAN	P62987	Ubiquitin-ribosomal protein eL40 fusion protein	128	0	4	2.107474
ARP2_HUMAN	P61160	Actin-related protein 2	394	0	4	2.107474
BMS1_HUMAN	Q14692	Ribosome biogenesis protein BMS1 homolog	1282	0	4	2.107474

4. Discussion

Previous research has shown that the prevalence of NUCs, graded at level ≥1 according to the WHO cataract grading system, was notably higher in tropical and subtropical regions than in temperate and subarctic regions regardless of racial factors [5–7]. In addition, it was reported that cumulative heat exposure is positively corelated with NUC incidence when the lens temperature exceeds 37.5 °C [5,10]. Thus, elevated lens temperatures resulting from higher environmental temperatures may contribute to an increased risk of NUC formation. However, the exact connection between NUCs and temperature is yet to be fully understood. We demonstrated the types of proteins expressed under normal and warming conditions by using shotgun proteomic analysis and found a decrease in the specific proteins involved in actin, tubulin, ubiquitin, ribosome, and histone under warming conditions in this study.

First, we determined the incubation temperature at normal-temp and warming-temp following a previous computer simulation in silico study [14] and identified 30 proteins exhibiting > 2-fold changes in expression between iHLEC-NY2 under normal-temp and warming-temp. Furthermore, the effect on the expression system is typically more significant when a protein is underexpressed compared to when it is overexpressed. Therefore, we have focused on variations in the expression of 11 factors (the specific proteins concerned were actin, tubulin, ubiquitin, ribosome, and histone), as described in Table 6. Decreased actin and tubulin expression was observed under warming conditions (Table 1). The cytoskeleton of the human eye, comprising actin microfilaments, intermediate filaments, microtubules, and their associated proteins, is essential for cellular growth, maturation, differentiation, integrity, and function. Actin microfilaments are composed of F-actin helices, which are built from G-actin subunits (47 kD) [23,24]. These filaments are distributed throughout the cytoplasm, form a fine mesh under the plasma membrane, or organize into stress fibers. The processes of actin polymerization and depolymerization are modulated by actin-regulatory proteins such as gelsolin. Additionally, various associated proteins bind actin filaments to the plasma membrane, supporting the cellular architecture [23,24]. Therefore, a decrease in actin levels may weaken cell membrane protein binding, resulting in lens opacity.

The putative tubulin-like protein alpha-4B is a cytoskeletal protein that constitutes a part of a structure known as microtubules. Microtubules play a crucial role in maintaining cell shape, cell division, and intracellular transport. Tubulin forms microtubules by dimerizing α-tubulin and β-tubulin, thereby providing structural stability within cells. The lens cells rely on microtubules to maintain their morphology [25]. Tubulin dysfunction can compromise microtubule stability, thus leading to alterations in cell shape and function, which may result in the loss of lens transparency. Furthermore, microtubules are essential for the proper transport of proteins within cells, including lens cells, where their functions are critical [26]. Abnormalities in putative tubulin-like protein alpha-4B may disrupt protein transport, potentially causing protein aggregation within the lens. This aggregation contributes to lens opacification. Additionally, because microtubules are involved in the proliferation and maintenance of lens cells, tubulin defects can lead to cellular dysfunction, which may contribute to lens opacity. Therefore, the putative tubulin-like protein alpha-4B plays a vital role in maintaining the structural integrity of lens cells and protein transport. A reduction in putative tubulin-like protein alpha-4B under high-temperature conditions may be one of the factors that contribute to lens opacification.

In addition, the expression of the proteins related to ubiquitin and ribosome in warming-temp-incubated iHLEC-NY2 was also lower than that in normal-temp-incubated iHLEC-NY2. Many of the signals that maintain lens epithelia appear to be substrates of the ubiquitin–proteasome pathway [27]. Ubiquitin C-terminal hydrolase L17-like protein 1 is an enzyme that is responsible for protein degradation and is particularly involved in the ubiquitin–proteasome system, a key protein quality control mechanism [28,29]. This system is essential for preserving cellular homeostasis by facilitating the elimination of damaged or misfolded proteins.

The eL40 fusion protein consists of ubiquitin, which tags damaged or unnecessary proteins for degradation, and the ribosomal protein eL40, which is involved in protein synthesis [30]. The BMS1 homolog is crucial for ribosome assembly, particularly ribosomal RNA (rRNA) processing and ribosomal subunit assembly [31]. Ribosomes are essential for protein synthesis within cells, and proteins such as BMS1 are indispensable for the proper formation of functional ribosomes [32]. Impairment of ribosome biogenesis can lead to increased production of misfolded proteins, especially in long-lived cells such as lens cells, which can contribute to cataract formation. Therefore, dysfunctions or mutations in BMS1 may increase the risk of cataract development.

Histones are key proteins involved in DNA packaging within the nuclei of eukaryotic cells. They wrap DNA to form chromatin, thus enabling it to be compactly stored and to regulate gene expression [33]. If histone modifications or structural changes adversely affect the expression of genes that are critical for maintaining lens transparency, improper protein folding and aggregation within the lens may occur, leading to loss of lens transparency.

Moreover, we examined their functions by analyzing the four GO terms (Tables 1–4). The GO analysis indicated that the most common factors identified in the molecular function, cellular component, biological processes, and KEGG pathway categories were "protein binding", "extracellular exosome", "nucleosome assembly", and "neutrophil extracellular trap formation", respectively (Tables 1–4). The proteins involved in protein binding were actin and alpha cardiac muscle 1. The proteins associated with extracellular exosomes included actin, alpha cardiac muscle 1, actin-related protein 2, ribosome biogenesis protein BMS1 homolog, histone H2B type 1-M, and histone H2B type 1-M. Additionally, the protein involved in nucleosome assembly was histone H2B type 1-M. Taken together, it is possible that factors associated with actin, ribosomes, and histones are specifically involved in the onset of cataracts due to temperature changes. However, the present results also show that the expression of other proteins related to tubulin and histones, such as tubulin alpha-1C chain and histone-H2B type 1-C/E/F/G/I, -H2B type F-S, -H2B type 1-D, -H2A type 1-H, and -H3.1, increases at warming-temp (Table 5). Therefore, changes in the tubulin and histone levels may be associated with homeostatic maintenance. Further investigations are required in order to determine whether the decrease or increase in these proteins at higher ambient temperatures plays a dominant role.

It is crucial to explore whether the overexpression of certain proteins and the reduction in others at elevated temperatures are associated with lens dysfunction. In our previous study utilizing a similar shotgun proteomic analysis, we demonstrated that heating the rat whole lens (including the epithelium, cortex, and nucleus) at warming-temp resulted in reductions in actin, tubulin, vimentin, filensin, and fatty acid-binding protein 5 [11]. Among these, both actin and tubulin were found to decrease upon heating in both the rat lens and iHLEC-NY2. These findings suggest that the observed reductions in actin and tubulin may at least be attributable to epithelial cells. Thus, this study has successfully screened lens proteins that change in response to elevated temperature, which were previously unidentified as potential causes of NUCs. As a result, it is now possible to consider temperature-related factors in NUC development, contributing to future research advancements. However, this study does not fully reflect the changes occurring in the nuclear or cortical regions of the lens since human epithelial cells were used. Moreover, additional research is required to assess the relationship between the onset of NUCs and changes in the proteins involved in actin, tubulin, ubiquitin, ribosomes, and histones. Therefore, we are planning to measure the localization and expression of the specific proteins concerning actin, tubulin, ubiquitin, ribosomes, and histones under warming-temp by using Western blotting and an immunostaining method.

5. Conclusions

The conducted shotgun proteomic analysis revealed that warming decreased the expression of specific proteins involved in actin, tubulin, ubiquitin, ribosomes, and histones in iHLEC-NY2. This study could provide a valuable framework for understanding the relationship between temperature and the onset of NUCs. However, additional research is necessary to fully comprehend the mechanisms that link these factors. In addition, regarding the clinical correlation of shotgun proteomics and future directions, it is desirable to investigate whether similar protein fluctuations occur using postoperative samples from human NUC patients. Furthermore, establishing prevention or treatment strategies for nuclear cataracts by suppressing these protein fluctuations is anticipated.

Author Contributions: Conceptualization, H.O. and N.N.; methodology, H.O., A.T., H.S. and N.N.; formal analysis, H.O., T.Y., N.Y., Y.N., Y.M. and A.T.; investigation, H.O., T.Y., N.Y., Y.N., Y.M. and H.S.; data curation, H.O., T.Y., A.T. and H.S.; writing—original draft preparation, H.O. and N.N.; writing—review and editing, H.O. and N.N.; visualization, N.N.; supervision, N.N.; funding acquisition, N.N. All authors have read and agreed to the published version of the manuscript.

Funding: This research was funded by Takeda Science Foundation Pharmaceutical Research Grants (grant number: 2024068087).

Institutional Review Board Statement: This study was approved by the Ethics Review Committee of Fujita Health University (No. 004, approval date 1 April 2021) and was conducted in accordance with the provisions of the Declaration of Helsinki for research involving human tissue. This gene-recombination experiment was approved by the Kanazawa Medical University Biosafety Committee for Recombinant DNA Research (Approval No. 2020-18, approval date 11 November 2020).

Informed Consent Statement: Not applicable.

Data Availability Statement: The raw MS data files were deposited in the ProteomeXchange Consortium via the jPOST partner repository (http://jpostdb.org, accessed on 18 January 2025) under the dataset identifier PXD059029/JPST003507. Publicly available datasets, such as the UniProt dataset (https://www.uniprot.org/help/downloads, accessed on 18 January 2025) utilized in this study, can also be accessed through their respective repositories following the guidelines provided by the data-sharing platforms. The data generated in this study can be requested from the corresponding author.

Conflicts of Interest: The authors declare no conflicts of interest.

Abbreviations

DAVID	Database for Annotation, Visualization, and Integrated Discovery
GO	Gene Ontology
KEGG	Kyoto Encyclopedia of Genes and Genomes
LC–MS/MS	Liquid chromatography with tandem mass spectrometry
NSAF	Normalized spectral abundance factor
NSI	Nanoelectrospray ionization
NUC	Nuclear cataract
Rsc	log2-transformed ratio of protein abundances

References

1. Robman, L.; Taylor, H. External factors in the development of cataract. *Eye* **2005**, *19*, 1074–1082. [CrossRef] [PubMed]
2. Chua, J.; Koh, J.Y.; Tan, A.G.; Zhao, W.; Lamoureux, E.; Mitchell, P.; Wang, J.J.; Wong, T.Y.; Cheng, C.-Y. Ancestry, Socioeconomic Status, and Age-Related Cataract in Asians: The Singapore Epidemiology of Eye Diseases Study. *Ophthalmology* **2015**, *122*, 2169–2178. [CrossRef] [PubMed]
3. Kai, J.-Y.; Zhou, M.; Li, D.-L.; Zhu, K.-Y.; Wu, Q.; Zhang, X.-F.; Pan, C.-W. Smoking, dietary factors and major age-related eye disorders: An umbrella review of systematic reviews and meta-analyses. *Br. J. Ophthalmol.* **2023**, *108*, 51–57. [CrossRef] [PubMed]
4. Xu, Y.; Liang, A.; Zheng, X.; Huang, Z.; Li, Q.; Su, T.; Wu, Q.; Fang, Y.; Hu, Y.; Sun, W.; et al. Sex-specific social, lifestyle, and physical health risk factors in cataracts development. *Eye* **2024**, *38*, 2939–2946. [CrossRef]
5. Sasaki, K.; Sasaki, H.; Jonasson, F.; Kojima, M.; Cheng, H.M. Racial differences of lens transparency properties with aging and prevalence of age related cataract applying a WHO classification system. *Ophthalmic. Res.* **2004**, *36*, 332–340. [CrossRef] [PubMed]

6. Miyashita, H.; Hatsusaka, N.; Shibuya, E.; Mita, N.; Yamazaki, M.; Shibata, T.; Ishida, H.; Ukai, Y.; Kubo, E.; Sasaki, H. Association between ultraviolet radiation exposure dose and cataract in Han people living in China and Taiwan: A cross sectional study. *PLoS ONE* **2019**, *14*, e0215338.
7. Sasaki, H.; Jonasson, F.; Shui, Y.B.; Kojima, M.; Ono, M.; Katoh, N.; Cheng, H.-M.; Takahashi, N.; Sasaki, K. High prevalence of nuclear cataract in the population of tropical and subtropical areas. *Dev. Ophthalmol.* **2002**, *35*, 60–69. [PubMed]
8. Al-Ghadyan, A.A.; Cotlier, E. Rise in lens temperature on exposure to sunlight or high ambient temperature. *Br. J. Ophthalmol.* **1986**, *70*, 421–426. [CrossRef] [PubMed]
9. Schwartz, B. Environmental temperature and the ocular temperature gradient. *Arch. Ophthalmol.* **1965**, *74*, 237–243. [CrossRef]
10. Kodera, S.; Hirata, A.; Miura, F.; Rashed, E.A.; Hatsusaka, N.; Yamamoto, N.; Kudo, E.; Sasaki, H. Model-based approach for analyzing prevalence of nuclear cataracts in elderly residents. *Comput. Biol. Med.* **2020**, *126*, 104009. [CrossRef] [PubMed]
11. Otake, H.; Masuda, S.; Yamamoto, T.; Miyata, Y.; Nakazawa, Y.; Yamamoto, N.; Taga, A.; Sasaki, H.; Nagai, N. Semiquantitative analysis of protein expression in heated rat lens using shotgun proteomics. *Mol. Med. Rep.* **2025**, *31*, 26. [CrossRef]
12. Joseph, R.; Srivastava, O.P.; Pfister, R.R. Differential epithelial and stromal protein profiles in keratoconus and normal human corneas. *Exp. Eye Res.* **2011**, *92*, 282–298. [CrossRef] [PubMed]
13. Meade, M.L.; Shiyanov, P.; Schlager, J.J. Nhanced detection ethod for corneal protein identification using shotgun roteomics. *Proteome Sci.* **2009**, *7*, 23. [CrossRef] [PubMed]
14. Takeda, S.; Yamamoto, N.; Nagai, N.; Hiramatsu, N.; Deguchi, S.; Hatsusaka, N.; Kubo, E.; Sasaki, H. Function of mitochondrial cytochrome c oxidase is enhanced in human lens epithelial cells at high temperatures. *Mol. Med. Rep.* **2023**, *27*, 19. [CrossRef] [PubMed]
15. Yamasaki, K.; Kawasaki, S.; Young, R.D.; Fukuoka, H.; Tanioka, H.; Nakatsukasa, M.; Quantock, A.J.; Kinoshita, S. Genomic aberrations and cellular heterogeneity in SV40-immortalized human corneal epithelial cells. *Investig. Ophthalmol. Vis. Sci.* **2009**, *50*, 604–613. [CrossRef]
16. Kim, C.W.; Go, R.E.; Lee, G.A.; Kim, C.D.; Chun, Y.J.; Choi, K.C. Immortalization of human corneal epithelial cells using simian virus 40 large T antigen and cell characterization. *J. Pharmacol. Toxicol. Methods* **2016**, *78*, 52–57. [CrossRef]
17. Bluemlein, K.; Ralser, M. Monitoring protein expression in whole cell extracts by targeted label- and standard-free LC-MS/MS. *Nat. Protoc.* **2011**, *6*, 859–869. [CrossRef] [PubMed]
18. Old, W.M.; Meyer-Arendt, K.; Aveline-Wolf, L.; Pierce, K.G.; Mendoza, A.; Sevinsky, J.R.; Resing, K.A.; Ahn, N.G. Comparison of label free methods for quantifying human proteins by shotgun proteomics. *Mol. Cell. Proteom.* **2005**, *4*, 1487–1502. [CrossRef] [PubMed]
19. Zybailov, B.; Coleman, M.K.; Florens, L.; Washburn, M.P. Correlation of relative adundance ratios derived from peptide ion chromatograms and spectrum counting for quantitative proteomic analysis using stable isotope labeling. *Anal. Chem.* **2005**, *77*, 6218–6224. [CrossRef]
20. Dennis, G., Jr.; Sherman, B.T.; Hosack, D.A.; Yang, J.; Gao, W.; Lane, H.C.; Lempicki, R.A. DAVID: Database for annotation, visualization, and integrated discovery. *Genome Biol.* **2003**, *4*, R60. [CrossRef]
21. Huang, D.W.; Sherman, B.T.; Lempicki, R.A. Systematic and integrative analysis of large gene lists using DAVID bioinformatics resources. *Nat. Protoc.* **2009**, *4*, 44–57. [CrossRef] [PubMed]
22. Huang, D.W.; Sherman, B.T.; Zheng, X.; Yang, J.; Inamichi, T.; Stephens, R.; Lempicki, R.A. Extracting biological meaning from large gene lists with DAVID. *Curr. Protoc. Bioinform.* **2009**, *27*, 13.11.1–13.11.13. [CrossRef]
23. Weeds, A.G.; Gooch, J.; Hawkins, M.; Pops, B.; Way, M. Role of actin-binding proteins in cytoskeletal dynamics. *Biochem. Soc. Trans.* **1991**, *19*, 1016–1020. [CrossRef] [PubMed]
24. Kivelä, T.; Tarkkanen, A.; Frangione, B.; Ghiso, J.; Haltia, M. Ocular amyloid deposition in familial amyloidosis, Finnish: An analysis of native and variant gelsolin in Meretoja's syndrome. *Investig. Ophthalmol. Vis. Sci.* **1994**, *35*, 3759–3769.
25. Farnsworth, P.N.; Shybe, S.E.; Caputo, S.J.; Fasano, A.V.; Spector, A. Microtubules: A major cytoskeletal component of the human lens. *Exp. Eye Res.* **1980**, *30*, 611–615. [CrossRef] [PubMed]
26. Audette, D.S.; Scheiblin, D.A.; Duncan, M.K. The molecular mechanisms underlying lens fiber elongation. *Exp. Eye Res.* **2017**, *156*, 41–49. [CrossRef] [PubMed]
27. Roberts, A.B.; Derynck, R. Meeting report: Signaling schemes for TGF-beta. *Sci. STKE* **2001**, *113*, pe43.
28. Nagasaka, M.; Inoue, Y.; Yoshida, M.; Miyajima, C.; Morishita, D.; Tokugawa, M.; Nakamoto, H.; Sugano, M.; Ohoka, N.; Hayashi, H. The deubiquitinating enzyme USP17 regulates c-Myc levels and controls cell proliferation and glycolysis. *FEBS Lett.* **2022**, *596*, 465–478. [CrossRef] [PubMed]
29. Ramakrishna, S.; Suresh, B.; Baek, K.-H. Biological functions of hyaluronan and cytokine-inducible deubiquitinating enzymes. *Biochim. Biophys. Acta* **2015**, *1855*, 83–91. [CrossRef] [PubMed]
30. Tong, L.; Zheng, X.; Wang, T.; Gu, W.; Shen, T.; Yuan, W.; Wang, S.; Xing, S.; Liu, X.; Zhang, C.; et al. Inhibition of UBA52 induces autophagy via EMC6 to suppress hepatocellular carcinoma tumorigenesis and progression. *J. Cell. Mol. Med.* **2024**, *28*, e18164. [CrossRef]

31. Singh, S.; Broeck, A.V.; Miller, L.; Chaker-Margot, M.; Klinge, S. Nucleolar maturation of the human small subunit processome. *Science* **2021**, *373*, eabj5338. [CrossRef]
32. Karbstein, K.; Jonas, S.; Doudna, J.A. An essential GTPase promotes assembly of preribosomal RNA processing complexes. *Mol. Cell* **2005**, *20*, 633–643. [CrossRef]
33. Andley, U.P.; Naumann, B.N.; Hamilton, P.D.; Bozeman, S.L. Changes in relative histone abundance and heterochromatin in αA-crystallin and αB-crystallin knock-in mutant mouse lenses. *BMC Res. Notes* **2020**, *13*, 315. [CrossRef]

medicina

MDPI

Article

Disinfection of Human and Porcine Corneal Endothelial Cells by Far-UVC Irradiation

Ben Sicks [1,*], Martin Hessling [1], Kathrin Stucke-Straub [1], Sebastian Kupferschmid [2] and Ramin Lotfi [3]

1 Institute of Medical Engineering and Mechatronics, Ulm University of Applied Sciences, Albert-Einstein-Allee 55, 89081 Ulm, Germany; martin.hessling@thu.de (M.H.); kathrin.stucke-straub@thu.de (K.S.-S.)
2 Clinic of Ophthalmology, Bundeswehrkrankenhaus Ulm, Oberer Eselsberg 40, 89081 Ulm, Germany; sebastiankupferschmid@bundeswehr.org
3 Institute for Clinical Transfusion Medicine and Immunogenetics Ulm, German Red Cross Blood Donation Service Baden-Württemberg-Hessen, Institute for Transfusion Medicine, University Hospital Ulm, Helmholtzstraße 10, 89081 Ulm, Germany; r.lotfi@blutspende.de
* Correspondence: ben.sicks@thu.de

Abstract: *Background and Objectives*: The cornea protects the eye from external influences and contributes to its refractive power. Corneas belong to the most frequently transplanted tissues, providing a last resort for preserving the patient's vision. There is a high demand for donor corneas worldwide, but almost 4% of these transplants are not eligible due to microbial contamination. The objective of this study is to ascertain the suitability of 222 nm Far-UVC irradiation for the decontamination of corneas without damaging corneal endothelial cells. *Materials and Methods*: To assess the destructive effect of irradiation and, thus, identify the applicable dose needed to decontaminate the cornea without interfering with its integrity, 141 porcine corneas were irradiated with 0, 60 or 150 mJ/cm^2 at 222 nm. In the second step, a series of 13 human corneas were subjected to half-sided irradiation using 15 or 60 mJ/cm^2 at 222 nm. After five days of in vitro culturing, the endothelial cell density of the non-irradiated area of each human cornea was compared to the irradiated area. *Results*: Irradiation with up to 60 mJ/cm^2 had no detectably significant effect on the cell integrity of human corneas ($p = 0.764$), with only a minimal reduction in cell density of 3.7% observed. These findings were partially corroborated by tests on porcine corneas, wherein the variability between test groups was consistent, even at increased irradiation doses of up to 150 mJ/cm^2, and no notable effects on the irradiated porcine endothelium were monitored. The efficacy of the antimicrobial treatment was evident in the disinfection tests conducted on corneas. *Conclusions*: These initial irradiation experiments demonstrated that 222 nm Far-UVC radiation has the potential to decontaminate the cornea without compromising sensitive endothelial cell viability.

Keywords: cornea irradiation; donor; transplant; human eye; 222 nm Far-UVC

1. Introduction

Corneas are commonly known as the visual gateway to the world due to their optical properties [1,2]. Various serious diseases or injuries, which impact corneal integrity, can lead to vision loss [3–7]. In such cases, keratoplasty is often considered as the last option to save eyesight. Annually, over 200,000 corneas are transplanted worldwide [8]. For a keratoplasty, donor corneas are needed, which must fulfil various quality criteria [9]. Corneal transplants need to be free of pathogens and to have a sufficient density of endothelial cells [10]. Corneal endothelial cells (CECs) are in charge of maintaining corneal clarity by preventing the cornea from becoming edematous [11,12]. Unfortunately, CECs are very sensitive to chemical and physical stress and do not have regenerative capacities, which leads to the continuous loss of their number during life span [1,11,13,14]. This results in the exclusion of a considerable proportion of tissue donations not fulfilling minimal criteria for endothelial cell density. In addition, bacterial contamination occurs in some donations, which, in turn, leads to further exclusion of donor tissues. About 9% of all cultured corneas in Germany have to be discharged due to contamination [15].

Far-UVC, with a spectral range of 200–230 nm [16], exhibits strong antimicrobial properties similar to the antimicrobial properties at 254 nm UVC radiation, based on DNA and RNA absorption [17]. Far-UVC is also absorbed by proteins, which largely shield the nucleus in irradiated mammalian cells [18,19]. Studies have shown that Far-UVC doses up to 600 mJ/cm^2 are harmless to the outer corneal layers, while a dose of 15 mJ/cm^2 is sufficient for a 3 log reduction in methicillin-resistant *Staphylococcus aureus* (*S. aureus*) (MRSA) [20–23]. The American Conference of Governmental Industrial Hygienists (ACGIH) sets the safe exposure limit for eyes to 222 nm Far-UVC irradiation at 167.6 mJ/cm^2 [24].

The hCorneas are retrieved from deceased donors in a sterile environment, following strict eye bank protocols to preserve sterility and tissue viability while minimizing damage during dissection [25]. After extraction, corneas are disinfected to eliminate pathogens, typically by immersion in 3% povidone-iodine, followed by saline rinsing [26]. In addition, atmospheric-pressure cold plasma (APCP) has been explored as an alternative disinfection method, effectively inactivating pathogens without compromising tissue integrity [27]. For xenotransplantation, the extraction of porcine corneas typically begins with anesthesia to ensure the animal remains still and pain-free [28]. The eyes are then enucleated in a sterile environment to prevent contamination, followed by precise dissection of the cornea to minimize tissue damage [29]. Once extracted, the corneas are preserved in an appropriate medium to maintain viability for research or transplantation purposes [30].

The objective of this study is to determine the appropriate disinfecting dose of 222 nm Far-UVC radiation that can be tolerated by CECs while being sufficient to induce decontamination. For this purpose, the human corneal endothelial cells (hCECs) of cultured human corneas (hCorneas) are irradiated with up to 60 mJ/cm^2, cultured again, and the cell density is recorded at regular intervals. A set of cultured corneas is used to compare the behavior during recultivation after irradiation. Furthermore, pairs of eyes from the same donor are subjected to an investigation to ascertain the existence of any potential correlations. Experiments on porcine corneas (pCorneas) at irradiation doses of up to 150 mJ/cm^2 on porcine corneal endothelial cells (pCECs) provide supplementary evidence. The results are subjected to statistical evaluation.

2. Materials and Methods

The pCorneas used in this study were obtained from freshly slaughtered pigs. The corneas were extracted from the bulbi in a sterile laboratory environment. Prior to extraction, the bulbi were disinfected in a 2% iodine solution for three to five minutes and subsequently washed in sterile balanced salt solution (BSS). Extraction was performed by cutting along the scleral rim. The extracted corneal disc was temporarily stored in sterile phosphate-buffered saline (PBS).

The hCorneas were provided by the tissue bank IKT (Institute for Clinical Transfusion Medicine and Immunogenetics) Ulm, Germany. The cell densities at the beginning and end of the cultivation process were recorded. A set comprising corneas routinely cultivated in the tissue bank was employed to assess the normal performance of the corneas during cultivation and to ascertain the independence of two corneas from the same donor.

The corneas of humans and pigs are structurally similar in diameter (10–12 mm vs. 12–14 mm) and thickness (550–700 μm vs. 666–1013 μm). There is a similarity in the density of CECs (2500–4000 cells/mm^2 in the hCorneas and 3250–4411 cells/mm^2 in the pCorneas) and in the layers (epithelium, Bowman's membrane, stroma, Descement's membrane and endothelium) [13,29,31]. The mechanical properties are comparable in tensile strength and stress–strain relationships under uniaxial testing, but there are significant differences in stress relaxation [30]. The pCECs recover or regenerate more than hCECs, which mostly do not. This characteristic contributes to the resilience of pCECs for transplantation, making it more likely that, with appropriate therapy, porcine tissues can be applied in medical treatments [29]. The probability of an immune response arising from Far-UVC exposure to the endothelium is negligible because the primary objective is to avert any potential damage to the CECs.

The irradiation setup used a krypton chloride excimer lamp (Care222®, Ushio, Tokyo, Japan), and an X1 optometer (Gigahertz-Optik, Türkenfeld, Germany) was used to set an irradiance of 1 mW/cm^2. The cornea was fixed in a Böhnke holder within an empty modified cell culture flask with a window for the irradiated area (Figure 1). The concave side of the cornea with the CECs was irradiated, in comparison to other tests (given that the cornea is not transparent at 222 nm [32–34]). In hCornea experiments, one half was irradiated, and the other served as control. To distinguish between sides, an incision was made at the scleral edge on each sample. The non-irradiation area was adequately covered. The pCECs were fully irradiated at doses of 60 and 150 mJ/cm^2 while hCECs received half-sided irradiation of 15 and 60 mJ/cm^2.

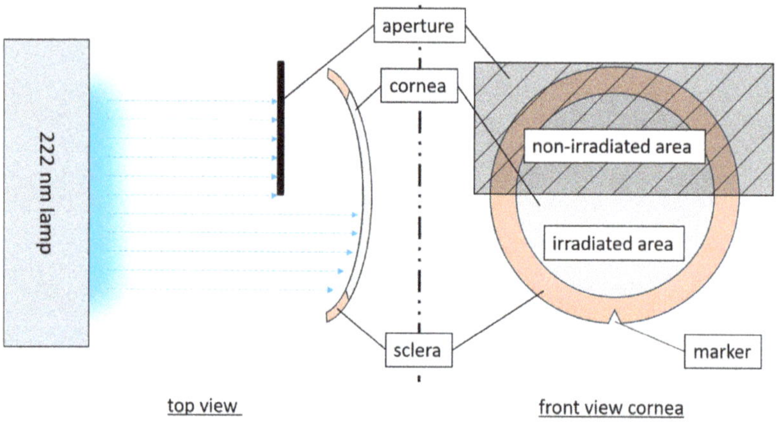

Figure 1. Schematic representation of the irradiation setup for hCornea with the partially blocked radiation pathway (top view) and the irradiation areas of a cornea (front view).

To examine the pCornea microscopically, an irradiated sample was trephined after a latency period of up to two hours. This corneal section was then stained. Viable CECs were evaluated and compared through staining in accordance with the instructions provided in the Viability/Cell toxicity Assay Kit for Animal Live & Dead cells (Biotium, Fremont, CA, USA) or with DAPI (4′,6-diamidino-2-phenylindole, dilactate) (Invitrogen, Carlsbad, CA, USA). An Eclipse TE2000-U (Nikon, Gyoda, Japan) fluorescence microscope was used to obtain multiple images of each cornea.

The integrity and density of the hCECs were determined via cell imaging prior to and immediately following irradiation, as well as at regular intervals up to the fifth day. Therefore, hCorneas were placed in a chamber of a 6-well plate, which was filled with 10 mL sterile PBS. At least five images of the hCECs per corneal half (irradiated/non-irradiated) were taken at each time of measurement with a phase contrast microscope (Primovert, Zeiss, Oberkochen, Germany) with 40× magnification.

The evaluation of pCECs and hCEC densities was carried out with ImageJ 1.53o [35] by creating a grid with a size of 0.1×0.1 mm^2 over the images to be analyzed. By using the CellCounter plugin [36], the cells of 4 fields were counted and averaged. This average was multiplied by one hundred to obtain cells/mm^2.

A disinfection test was conducted using *Staphylococcus carnosus* (DSM 20501) as a surrogate for *S. aureus*, given its comparable sensitivity to 222 nm UVC radiation [37]. A colony of *S. carnosus* was inoculated into 3 mL M92 medium and incubated at 37 °C for 16 h. Then, 200 µL of the preculture was transferred to 30 mL of fresh M92 medium and incubated at 37 °C until an optical density at 600 nm (OD_{600}) of 0.33 was reached. The culture was centrifuged and the supernatant replaced with PBS. This was repeated twice. The suspension was diluted to 10^7 colony-forming units (CFU) per milliliter. Disinfection tests were conducted on the concave side of pCorneas using two different thicknesses of bacterial suspension (1 mm and 3 mm) and three different Far-UVC doses (15, 60, and 150 mJ/cm^2). Following this, 33 µL samples were plated on M92 agar and incubated at 37 °C for 24 h to determine bacterial survival.

To analyze changes in cell density of hCECs over a five-day period, the cell density ratios (CDRs) were calculated by dividing the value of the last cell count by the value of the first cell count (Equation (1)) for each sample. It was assumed that a five-day observation period would be sufficient for the human corneas to show an effect on the sensitive endothelium.

$$cell\ density\ ratio\ (CDR) = \frac{cells/mm^2{}_{end\ of\ cultivation}}{cells/mm^2{}_{start\ of\ cultivation}}, \quad (1)$$

The relative change of cell counts (RCCC) was calculated by dividing CDR of irradiated side by CDR of non-irradiated side (Equation (2)).

$$RCCC = 1 - \frac{CDR_{irr}}{CDR_{non-irr}} = 1 - \frac{day5_{irr}/day1_{irr}}{day5_{non-irr}/day1_{non-irr}}, \quad (2)$$

Initial data analysis involved assessing normality using the Shapiro–Wilk test. To evaluate the homogeneity of variances, the Levene test was conducted. When variance homogeneity was confirmed, analysis of variance (ANOVA) with the F-test for multiple samples was performed. In the case of significant ANOVA results, the Bonferroni correction was applied to adjust the significance levels. If the data were not normally distributed, the Kruskal–Wallis test (H-test) was employed. For significant results from the Kruskal–Wallis test, Dunn's post hoc test was subsequently performed. A p-value of ≤ 0.05 was considered statistically significant. A Student's t-test for unpaired samples was conducted to ascertain the statistical significance of the observed differences. Analyses were performed using the statistical software R 4.2.1 [38].

Based on an assumed effect δ and standard deviation (SD), the sample size was determined in order to have 80% power (1-ß = 80% with a corresponding $z_{1-\beta}$-quantile of 0.84) for a significance level of 5% (corresponding $z_{1-\frac{\alpha}{2}}$-quantile of 1.96) using Equation (3) [39].

$$n = \left(z_{1-{}^{\alpha}/_{2}} + z_{1-\beta}\right)^2 * \frac{SD^2}{\delta^2}, \quad (3)$$

SD was calculated according to Equation (4). In order to calculate δ according to Equation (5), the initial test results were employed to derive the mean values.

$$SD = \sqrt{\frac{\sum(x-\overline{x})^2}{n-1}} \quad (4)$$

$$\delta = (\mu_1 - \mu_0) \tag{5}$$

A reference group (RG) was established for the purpose of determining normal behavior and for test size analysis. The reference data were based on 168 transplantable corneas from the tissue bank IKT Ulm.

The study size was calculated using the SD of the RG, as this group had sufficient values and represents normal behavior. The δ between the irradiated and non-irradiated corneal sides of initially irradiated hCornea samples was calculated and used.

$$SD_{RG} = \sqrt{\frac{\sum(x-\overline{x})^2}{n-1}} = 0.081 \tag{6}$$

$$\delta_{hC-sample} = (0.964 - 0.916) = 0.048 \tag{7}$$

$$n = (1.96 + 0.84)^2 * \frac{0.081^2}{0.048^2} = 22.3;\ n = 23 \tag{8}$$

The RG has an average hCEC density of 2510 cells/mm^2, with an SD of 244 cells/mm^2. By using a δ of 5% of the mean, a comparable sample size can be obtained:

$$n = (1.96 + 0.84)^2 * \frac{244^2}{125.5^2} = 29.6;\ n = 30 \tag{9}$$

3. Results

This study evaluated the applicability of an effective disinfection dose without compromising endothelial integrity.

The irradiation of the hCECs was conducted within a room exclusively designated for laboratory examinations. The removal times of the cornea from the culture medium or buffer were maintained as short as possible to ensure the preservation of tissue integrity, with only minor extensions being made to extend the removal times for the irradiation process. The porcine corneas were processed in a laboratory and subsequently handled with minimal exposure outside of the buffer. All experiments were conducted at room temperature and under aseptic conditions.

Irradiation was applied to the concave corneal side, the critical surface for donation, due to the endothelium's sensitivity and lack of regenerative capacity. The cornea's concave–convex shape led to slight inhomogeneity in surface irradiation; however, with central alignment, intensity variation remained within 0.08 mW/cm^2. At a lamp-sample distance of ~9 cm, no heating occurred.

3.1. *pCornea Results*

Staining results demonstrated accurate and clear cell nuclei in both DAPI and live–dead staining using fluorescence microscopy. There was no noticeable density thinning or consistent decrease in density. However, in DAPI detection, there were areas where no CECs were present, as shown in Figure 2a. The staining for live and dead CECs revealed damaged or dead CECs in these areas (Figure 2b). A comparison of the two staining methods revealed no significant deviation in either variance (p = 0.135) or mean (p = 0.115). These findings support the applicability of DAPI staining for determining cell density. Structured damage caused by processing during trephination and dying, such as furrows, tweezer marks, and other pressure points, was not included in the count (Figure 2e). Additionally, irregular accumulations of damaged CECs were occasionally observed, as illustrated in Figure 2b. The cell shapes and spacing of the stained CECs showed an equal and regular distribution (Figure 2a–d). The staining of pCECs after 222 nm irradiation up to 150 mJ/cm^2 did not lead to a loss of structural integrity.

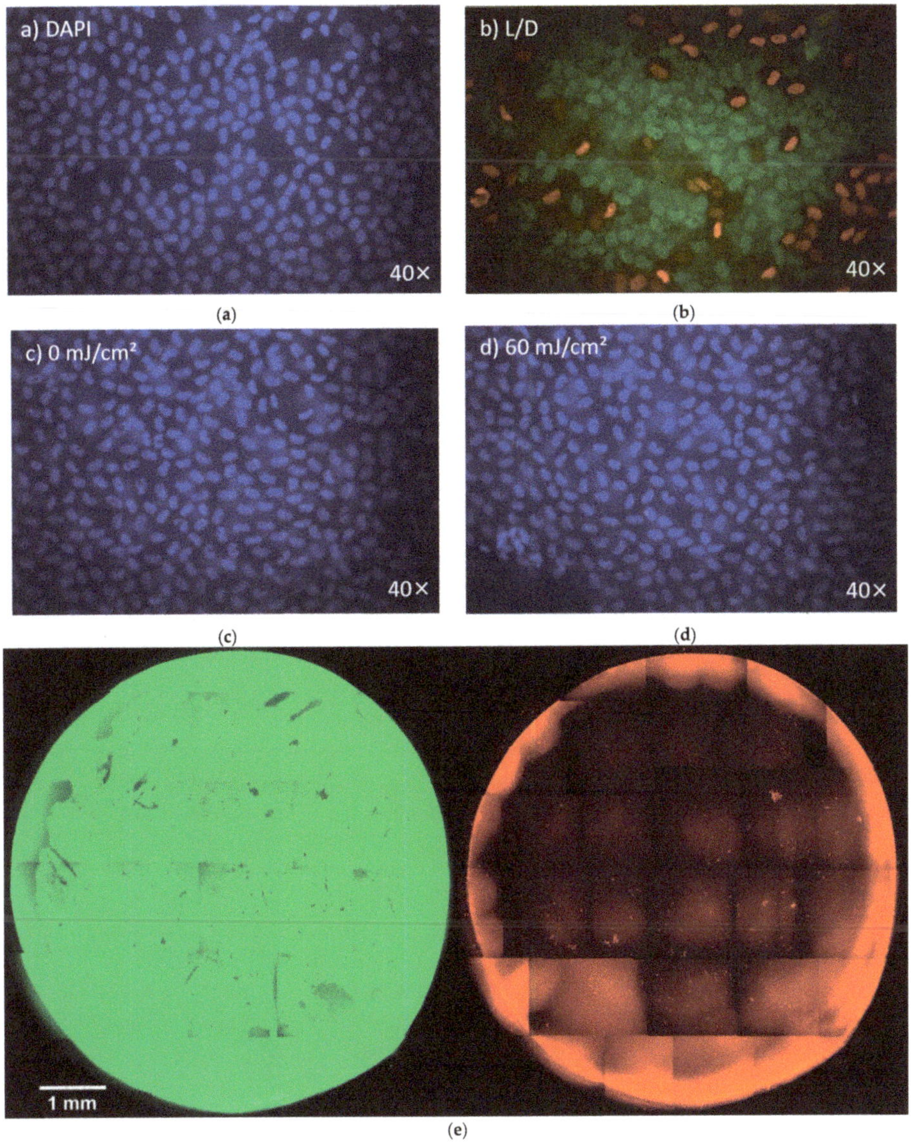

Figure 2. Comparison between a DAPI stain (**a**) and a live–dead stain (**b**); comparison between a non-irradiated (**c**) and 60 mJ/cm^2 irradiated endothelial layer after 2 days of cultivation. Images taken with a fluorescence microscope at 40× magnification (**d**). A disc of cornea was cut from a pCornea and stained with a live–dead dye. The two stains, live (left, green) and dead (right, red), are recorded separately from the same cornea. Images taken with a fluorescence microscope at 10× magnification and stitched together (**e**).

The irradiation tests revealed that the mean CEC densities of the irradiation groups listed in Table 1 are distributed from 3873 to 3414 cells/mm^2. The SDs are around 9%, with only a few outliers. None of the outliers are below 3000 cells/mm^2, but some are above 4500 cells/mm^2. These outliers were included due to their high CEC densities, which are still within the characteristic range [29].

Table 1. The pCEC densities after irradiation at 222 nm, divided into the applied irradiation dose.

Irradiation Dose [mJ/cm^2]	0	60	150
Mean CECs [cells/mm^2]	3798	3572	3601
SD [cells/mm^2]	337	320	335
Number of corneas	57	39	45

The box plots representing the groups are presented in Figure 3.

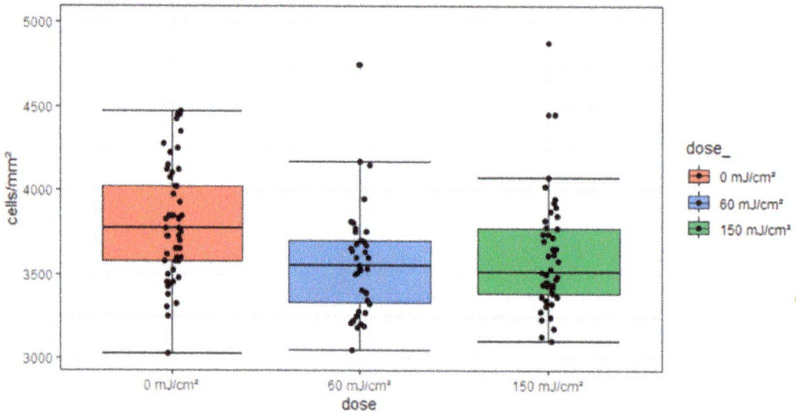

Figure 3. Dose-dependent grouping of pCEC densities from 222 nm irradiation.

In order to compare the three irradiation doses regarding the CEC densities, the Kruskal–Wallis test was applied since normality could not be assumed (demonstrated with Shapiro–Wilk test) and outliers are present in the sample. This Kruskal–Wallis test is more robust compared to a conventional ANOVA.

The Kruskal–Wallis test ($\chi^2(2) = 14.87$, $p < 0.001$) and post hoc tests demonstrated significant differences between the 0 mJ/cm^2 and 60 mJ/cm^2 groups and between the 0 mJ/cm^2 and 150 mJ/cm^2 groups.

The results of the microbiological (Figure 4) tests demonstrated that irradiation doses of 15 mJ/cm^2 achieved up to a 3-log reduction in microbial load within 1 mm thick liquid films. Furthermore, reductions of up to and over 5 log levels were achieved in 1 and 3 mm liquid layers with 60 mJ/cm^2.

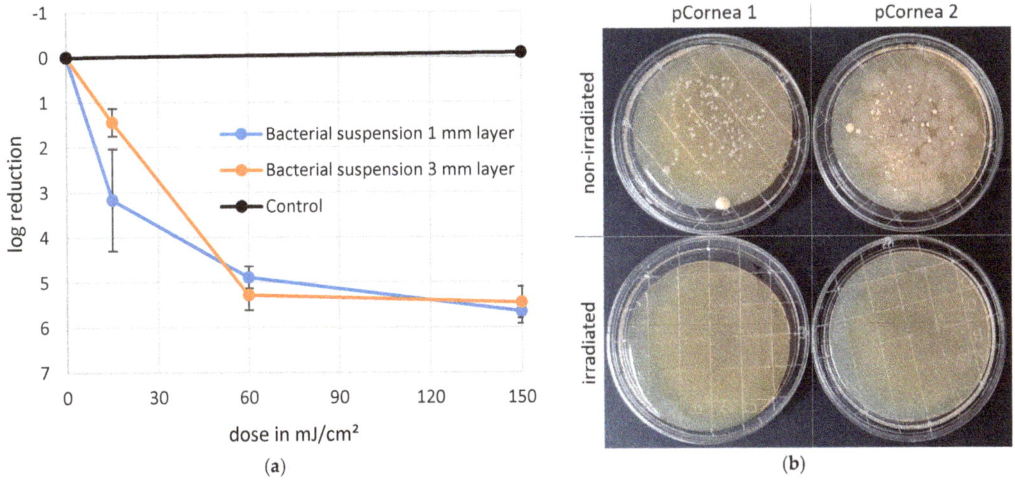

Figure 4. 222 nm disinfection of a one- and three-millimeter-thick layer of an *S. carnosus* bacterial suspension in a log-reduction graph (**a**) and a picture of contamination samples before and after irradiation plated on a tryptone soy agar plate to demonstrate the efficacy of the process (**b**).

3.2. hCornea Results

The mean hCEC density of the RG on the first day of culture was 2509 cells/mm^2 (SD = 243 cells/mm^2). On the last day (3 to 28 days later), the mean was 2338 cells/mm^2 (SD = 283 cells/mm^2). The mean CDR between the first and last day was 0.93 (SD = 0.081). Figure 5 presents all CDRs of the referenced data as a function of cultivation time, with a slightly decreasing straight line fit (CDR = $-0.0047x + 1$) (approx. 0.5% loss per day) for cultivation durations of 3 to 28 days (n = 168). The Shapiro–Wilk test was $p < 0.001$, indicating non-normal distribution of the CDRs, but the large sample size mitigates this issue for the regression model.

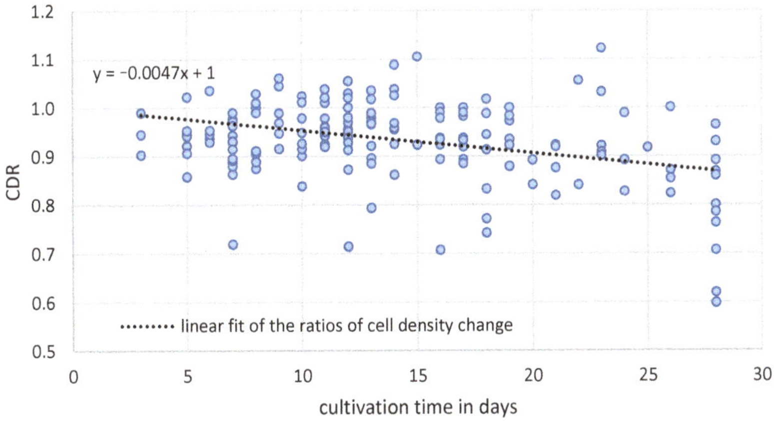

Figure 5. CDR values of the referenced group of the set of cultured corneas from the IKT Ulm, Germany.

Verification of the correlation between two corneas from the same donor: A total of 26 corneal pairs from the RG were analyzed, exhibiting a linear regression for the right/left ratio with a low coefficient of determination (R^2 = 0.0232) and no consistent or trend-like distribution of residuals. The regression lines for both corneal sides were parallel with a slight CDR offset of 0.025, indicating no significant difference in hCEC density behavior. A *t*-test confirmed this ($p = 0.491$).

Results of the irradiation tests: The normal incubation period of the corneas was five days, but one cornea was only incubated for three days as the quality of the hCECs deteriorated rapidly and could not be counted later. The hCEC densities from day five and the outlier from day three were used for statistical analysis. There was no visible change in the culture medium in any of the tests.

The CDR differences between the irradiation groups in Table 2, comprising irradiated vs. non-irradiated samples at each dose, resulted in a deviation of approximately 4.5% at 15 mJ/cm^2 and 5% at 60 mJ/cm^2. A two-sample *t*-test was conducted on the irradiation groups 15 ($p = 0.667$) and 60 mJ/cm^2 ($p = 0.582$), in which the CDR values of the non-irradiated corneal halves were compared against the corneal halves within the group. Nevertheless, no evidence of significance could be provided.

Table 2. The mean values ± SD of the results of the experiments with and without irradiation of hCECs, along with their CDRs (cell density ratios) of the cell densities from the day of irradiation and five days later, as well as the resulting RCCCs (relative change of cell counts).

		15 mJ/cm^2	60 mJ/cm^2	Σ
	n	5	8	13
Mean CEC counts for irradiated corneas ± standard deviation and cell density ratio (CDR)	day1	2405 ± 593	2028 ± 351	2173 ± 494
	day5	2205 ± 626	188 ± 521	2008 ± 585
	CDR	0.913	0.918	0.916
Mean CEC counts for non-irradiated corneas ± standard deviation and cell density ratio (CDR)	day1	2270 ± 450	1991 ± 350	2098 ± 414
	day5	2180 ± 539	1931 ± 511	2027 ± 535
	CDR	0.958	0.968	0.964
	RCCC	0.042	0.035	0.037

A comparison of the CDRs of the non-irradiated samples, designated "non-irradiated 15" and "non-irradiated 60", revealed no evidence for a statistically significant difference ($t(9) = -0.101$, $p = 0.922$). A corresponding calculation of the Cohen's d with the CDRs of the irradiation results indicated a tendency towards a small effect, with $d = 0.308$.

An ANOVA was conducted with the CDRs for each dose (0, 15, and 60 mJ/cm^2), revealing that the difference between the sample means of all groups in the comparison of irradiation application was not statistically significant ($F(2,23) = 0.273$, $p = 0.764$, $\eta^2 = 0.02$) (Figure 6, boxes on the right side). To assess the equality of variances, the Levene test was performed, which confirmed the assumption of equal variances ($p = 0.919$).

A further summary was conducted for the irradiated samples labelled 'irradiated 15' ($n = 5$) and 'irradiated 60' ($n = 8$), for which no statistically significant result could be demonstrated ($p = 0.954$). The data from the irradiated and non-irradiated samples were, therefore, summarized as 13 values each. A two-sample *t*-test of all irradiated and non-irradiated sample sides yielded a *p*-value of 0.462. These results suggest that the different doses did not have a measurable effect on the CDRs, indicating a lack of efficacy in this context.

Calculation of the RCCC, shown in Figure 7, and the cell count decrease between the first and the last day: The mean RCCC values were 0.042 for the 15 mJ/cm^2 group and 0.035 for the 60 mJ/cm^2 group, with an overall mean of 0.037. A *t*-test revealed no significant difference between the groups ($t(11) = 0.091$, $p = 0.929$, $\eta^2 = 0.056$, $d = 0.051$). Both groups were normally distributed (15 mJ/cm^2: $p = 0.531$, 60 mJ/cm^2: $p = 0.844$).

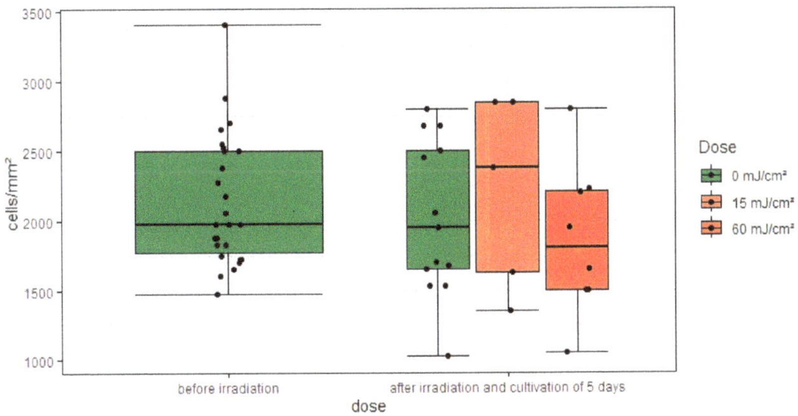

Figure 6. A grouped boxplot of the cell density depending on the irradiation dose.

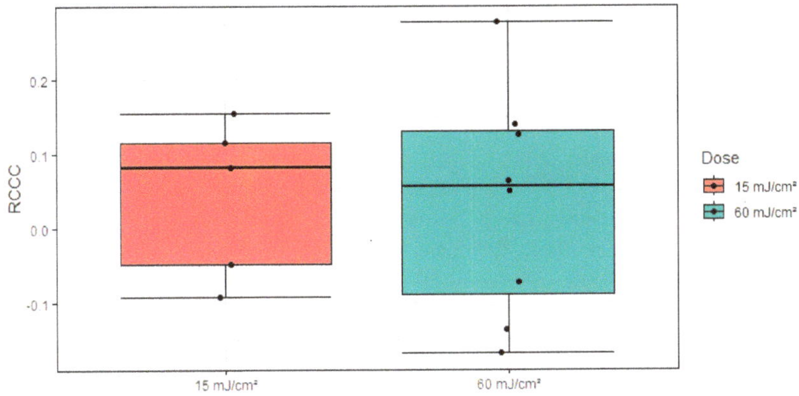

Figure 7. Boxplot of the RCCC values (dots) with the division into the irradiation groups 15 mJ/cm^2 (orange) and 60 mJ/cm^2 (blue).

4. Discussion

4.1. pCorneas

The CEC staining procedures did not yield any discernible alterations to the endothelium as a consequence of the radiation treatment. Consequently, any potential impairment in structural integrity can be ruled out.

The SD for the three test samples (0, 60 and 150 mJ/cm^2) was approximately 9%, indicating a similar degree of variability amongst the data points. The results of the Shapiro–Wilk test indicated that the 60 mJ/cm^2 and 150 mJ/cm^2 samples deviated from a normal distribution. Additionally, the groups exhibited outliers, making ANOVA insufficiently robust despite sufficient sample sizes of 57, 39, and 45. Therefore, the Kruskal–Wallis test was applied instead. The 60 and 150 mJ/cm^2 groups exhibited left skewness, likely due to outliers at high CEC densities, and resulted in a significant difference among the three samples. Nonetheless, the samples generally showed similar ranges, with means differing by less than 10%. Additionally, the evaluation did not indicate a significant difference in the applied exposures, suggesting a lack of effect rather than an actinic effect. However, further investigation is required into the impact of the effects on the subjects, as additional factors such as the animals' origins, handling of the subjects, and the processing of the subjects may also be contributing to the results.

Given the natural variability in CEC density among corneas, using a ratio metric such as the CDR or RCCC would have been more appropriate for analyzing and assessing the resulting cell densities post-irradiation with Far-UVC. This approach would have allowed for tracking changes in CEC density over time for each sample, facilitating better comparisons with other samples. Comparisons between hCECs and pCECs showed similar dispersion patterns and standard deviations.

The irradiation of the bacterial suspension on the endothelium was a relatively simple experimental setup, but it was quantitatively suboptimal. The high bacterial concentration on the endothelial surface represented an extreme case of microbial contamination, far from typical initial contamination levels. Nonetheless, the disinfection test clearly demonstrated the potential efficacy and application scope of this method.

4.2. *hCorneas*

The results of the paired comparisons suggest that a correlation between the CEC densities in the right and left corneas of a donor can be excluded and that all usable samples, including both corneas from the same donor, can be considered independent.

The CDR values of the entire reference group exhibit a regression pattern similar to that of the non-irradiated CECs in the test group during extended cultivation. The comparable slopes of the linear regressions in both groups suggest that their temporal behavior is nearly identical. The model indicates that while irradiation affects CEC density, this effect should be considered in the context of the normal cellular loss associated with cultivation.

The absence of a notable CDR test difference with the ANOVA test ($p = 0.767$) and the small effect size ($\eta^2 = 0.02$) lead to the conclusion that the irradiation is applicable. However, a significant alteration in CEC density could not be substantiated.

The relative difference in RCCC values between the two radiation doses of 0.007 is small compared to the mean value (0.037), as confirmed by a *t*-test ($p = 0.923$). The mean RCCC value of 0.037 corresponds to a 3.7% reduction in cell density in irradiated CECs compared to non-irradiated cells. This small effect size supports the hypothesis of a minimal radiation impact. It is important to note that the sample sizes for the RCCC groups ($n = 5$ and $n = 8$) are insufficient for precise study dimensioning but may be adequate for indicating trends.

4.3. *Overall*

Far-UVC at 222 nm has been shown to inactivate a wide range of bacteria, including those that are resistant to conventional antibiotics. This efficacy has also been demonstrated through the microbial test with S. carnosus as a surrogate for MRSA (see Figure 4) [37]. In contrast to conventional UVC, Far-UVC does not cause damage to cell nuclei or DNA due to its high protein absorption [40], making it a suitable method for surface disinfection and contamination control in clinical settings [41] on biological tissues and inorganic surfaces. However, certain limitations must be considered. Due to the shallow penetration depth of the radiation, its effectiveness is primarily restricted to surface disinfection or areas in close proximity to the exposure source. As a result, Far-UVC lacks the ability to penetrate deeper into tissues or complex structures, limiting its applicability in certain scenarios. These characteristics should be carefully evaluated when implementing this technology in clinical or industrial environments.

Due to the limited availability of hCorneas used in this study, the findings were supplemented by comparative investigations on porcine corneas. Although the initial results did not indicate any fundamental actinic changes in the CEC, it would be advisable to extend the studies on human corneas to the required sample size. Furthermore, additional studies should be conducted to obtain reliable conclusions. In particular, these should include investigations on the effects of increased radiation doses, assessments of cellular damage, and analyses of cellular changes following long-term incubation for up to 30 days.

On a structural level, there is similarity between human and porcine corneas. Combined with the apparent translatability, a similar response to environmental insults could be expected [29,30]. However, immunological disparities may influence responses to radiation, necessitating further investigation to assess their stability and suitability for exposure to radiation [29]. However, it is worth noting that the application of Far-UVC irradiation was limited to the CECs, because deeper tissue layers were not penetrated as the penetration depth was simply too low due to the high absorption [40].

5. Conclusions

Overall, no definitive conclusions could be drawn regarding the different test groups for porcine corneas due to excessive variance. The comparison based on cell densities without adjusting for individual variances proved problematic.

In contrast, when using CDR values and the resulting normalized values for human corneas, no significant effects from exposure to 222 nm radiation at doses up to 60 mJ/cm^2 were observed. This suggests that using 222 nm radiation for disinfection does not compromise the integrity of the endothelium, although it should be noted that the sample size was not sufficient for definitive conclusions. Further investigation into the threshold at which 222 nm radiation causes damage would be valuable. However, longer exposure times outside of a fluid buffer are unsuitable for the cornea. Irradiation within a non-absorbing buffer, such as PBS or BSS, could be considered.

Author Contributions: Conceptualization, S.K., M.H., B.S. and R.L.; methodology, M.H., B.S. and R.L.; validation, B.S. and R.L.; formal analysis, B.S., R.L. and K.S.-S.; investigation, B.S. and R.L.; resources, R.L. and M.H.; data curation, B.S.; writing—original draft preparation, B.S.; writing—review and editing, B.S., R.L., M.H., S.K. and K.S.-S.; visualization, B.S.; supervision, R.L., M.H. and S.K.; project administration, B.S.; funding acquisition, M.H. All authors have read and agreed to the published version of the manuscript.

Funding: This research received no external funding.

Institutional Review Board Statement: The study of human corneas was conducted in accordance with the Declaration of Helsinki and approved by the Ethics Committee of Universität Ulm (107/22, 27 May 2022). The study on pig corneas did not require ethical review and approval as the corneas were obtained from slaughtered animals sourced from a large slaughterhouse.

Informed Consent Statement: Not applicable.

Data Availability Statement: The original contributions presented in this study are included in the article. Further inquiries can be directed to the corresponding author.

Acknowledgments: The corneas were provided by the tissue bank IKT Ulm. Corneas were only used if they were not suitable for patient care because they did not fulfill the quality criteria a priori (e.g., endothelial cell density < 2000/mm^2) or showed a relevant quality loss during cultivation in the tissue bank IKT Ulm (i.e., >25% endothelial loss during cultivation).

Conflicts of Interest: The authors declare no conflicts of interest.

References

1. Eghrari, A.O.; Riazuddin, S.A.; Gottsch, J.D. Overview of the Cornea: Structure, Function, and Development. *Prog. Mol. Biol. Transl. Sci.* **2015**, *134*, 7–23. [CrossRef]
2. Sridhar, M.S. Anatomy of cornea and ocular surface. *Indian J. Ophthalmol.* **2018**, *66*, 190–194. [CrossRef]
3. Matthaei, M.; Sandhaeger, H.; Hermel, M.; Adler, W.; Jun, A.S.; Cursiefen, C.; Heindl, L.M. Changing Indications in Penetrating Keratoplasty: A Systematic Review of 34 Years of Global Reporting. *Transplantation* **2017**, *101*, 1387–1399. [CrossRef]

4. Whitcher, J.P.; Srinivasan, M.; Upadhyay, M.P. Corneal blindness: A global perspective. *Bull. World Health Organ.* **2001**, *79*, 214–221. [PubMed]
5. Green, M.; Apel, A.; Stapleton, F. Risk factors and causative organisms in microbial keratitis. *Cornea* **2008**, *27*, 22–27. [CrossRef] [PubMed]
6. Centers for Discease Control and Prevention. Basics of Bacterial Keratitis | Contact Lenses | CDC. Available online: https://www.cdc.gov/contact-lenses/causes/what-causes-contact-lens-related-bacterial-keratitis.html?CDC_AAref_Val=https://www.cdc.gov/contactlenses/bacterial-keratitis.html (accessed on 22 September 2021).
7. Rabinowitz, Y.S. Keratoconus. *Surv. Ophthalmol.* **1998**, *42*, 297–319. [CrossRef]
8. EBAA—Eye Bank Association of America. *2020 Eye Banking Statistical Report*; Eye Bank Association of America: Chantilly, VA, USA, 2021. Available online: https://restoresight.org/wp-content/uploads/2021/03/2020_Statistical_Report-Final.pdf (accessed on 10 November 2024).
9. EBAA. Eye Bank Association of America Medical Standards 2022: Eye Banking and Corneal Transplantation. *Eye Bank. Corneal Transplant.* **2022**, *1*, e002. [CrossRef]
10. Bundesärztekammer. Richtlinie zur Gewinnung von Spenderhornhäuten und zum Führen einer Augenhornhautbank, Erste Fortschreibung. *Dtsch. Arztebl.* **2018**, *115*, A262. Available online: https://www.bundesaerztekammer.de/fileadmin/user_upload/_old-files/downloads/pdf-Ordner/RL/Rili-Hornhaut.pdf (accessed on 5 February 2024).
11. Bonanno, J.A. Molecular mechanisms underlwordying the corneal endothelial pump. *Exp. Eye Res.* **2012**, *95*, 2–7. [CrossRef] [PubMed]
12. Cursiefen, C. *Immune Response and the Eye: Immune Privilege and Angiogenic Privilege of the Cornea*, 2nd ed.; Karger: Basel, Switzerland, 2007; Volume 92, pp. 50–57.
13. DelMonte, D.W.; Kim, T. Anatomy and physiology of the cornea. *J. Cataract Refract. Surg.* **2011**, *37*, 588–598. [CrossRef] [PubMed]
14. Adams, C.M.; Papillon, J.P.N.; Cioffi, C.L. (Eds.) *Drug Delivery Challenges and Novel Therapeutic Approaches for Retinal Diseases*; Springer: Cham, Switzerland, 2020; ISBN 978-3-030-56618-0.
15. Reinshagen, H.; Maier, P.C.; Böhringer, D. Aktivitäten der Sektion Gewebetransplantation und Biotechnologie der Deutschen Ophthalmologischen Gesellschaft: Leistungsbericht 2018. *Thieme Klin. Monatsbl. Augenheilkd.* **2021**, *238*, 186–190. [CrossRef]
16. International Ultraviolet Association. *Far UV-C Radiation: Current State-of Knowledge*; International Ultraviolet Association: Chevy Chase, MD, USA, 2021.
17. Bolton, J.R.; Cotton, C.A. *The Ultraviolet Disinfection Handbook*, 1st ed.; American Water Works Association: Denver, CO, USA, 2008; ISBN 9781613000779.
18. Coohill, T.P. Virus-cell interactions as probes for vacuum-ultraviolet radiation damage and repair. *Photochem. Photobiol.* **1986**, *44*, 359–363. [CrossRef]
19. Goldfarb, A.R.; Saidel, L.J. Ultraviolet absorption spectra of proteins. *Science* **1951**, *114*, 156–157. [CrossRef] [PubMed]
20. Kaidzu, S.; Sugihara, K.; Sasaki, M.; Nishiaki, A.; Igarashi, T.; Tanito, M. Evaluation of acute corneal damage induced by 222-nm and 254-nm ultraviolet light in Sprague-Dawley rats. *Free Radic. Res.* **2019**, *53*, 611–617. [CrossRef]
21. Ohashi, H.; Koi, T.; Igarashi, T. State-of-the-art Technology: Inactivation of Pathogens Using a 222-nm Ultraviolet Light Source with an Optical Filter. *J. Sci. Technol. Light.* **2021**, *44*, 9–11. [CrossRef]
22. Welch, D.; Aquino de Muro, M.; Buonanno, M.; Brenner, D.J. Wavelength-dependent DNA Photodamage in a 3-D human Skin Model over the Far-UVC and Germicidal UVC Wavelength Ranges from 215 to 255 nm. *Photochem. Photobiol.* **2022**, *98*, 1167–1171. [CrossRef] [PubMed]
23. Pitts, D.G.; Tredici, T.J. The effects of ultraviolet on the eye. *Am. Ind. Hyg. Assoc. J.* **1971**, *32*, 235–246. [CrossRef] [PubMed]
24. *TLVs® and BEIs®: Based on the Documentation of the Threshold Limit Values for Chemical Substances and Physical Agents & Biological Exposure Indices*; ACGIH: Cincinnati, OH, USA, 2022; ISBN 978-1-607261-52-0.
25. Armitage, W.J. Preservation of Human Cornea. *Transfus. Med. Hemother.* **2011**, *38*, 143–147. [CrossRef] [PubMed]
26. Kanavi, M.R.; Javadi, M.A.; Chamani, T.; Javadi, A. Screening of donated whole globes for photorefractive keratectomy. *Cornea* **2011**, *30*, 1260–1263. [CrossRef]
27. Brun, P.; Vono, M.; Venier, P.; Tarricone, E.; Deligianni, V.; Martines, E.; Zuin, M.; Spagnolo, S.; Cavazzana, R.; Cardin, R.; et al. Disinfection of ocular cells and tissues by atmospheric-pressure cold plasma. *PLoS ONE* **2012**, *7*, e33245. [CrossRef] [PubMed]
28. Faber, C.; Scherfig, E.; Prause, J.U.; Sørensen, K.E. Corneal Thickness in Pigs Measured by Ultrasound Pachymetry In Vivo. *Scand. J. Lab. Anim. Sci.* **2008**, *35*, 39–43.
29. Lee, S.E.; Mehra, R.; Fujita, M.; Roh, D.S.; Long, C.; Lee, W.; Funderburgh, J.L.; Ayares, D.L.; Cooper, D.K.C.; Hara, H. Characterization of porcine corneal endothelium for xenotransplantation. *Semin. Ophthalmol.* **2014**, *29*, 127–135. [CrossRef]
30. Hara, H.; Cooper, D.K.C. Xenotransplantation--the future of corneal transplantation? *Cornea* **2011**, *30*, 371–378. [CrossRef] [PubMed]
31. Sanchez, I.; Martin, R.; Ussa, F.; Fernandez-Bueno, I. The parameters of the porcine eyeball. *Graefes Arch. Clin. Exp. Ophthalmol.* **2011**, *249*, 475–482. [CrossRef] [PubMed]

32. Kaidzu, S.; Sugihara, K.; Sasaki, M.; Nishiaki, A.; Ohashi, H.; Igarashi, T.; Tanito, M. Re-Evaluation of Rat Corneal Damage by Short Wavelength UV Revealed Extremely Less Hazardous Property of Far-UV-C. *Photochem. Photobiol.* **2021**, *97*, 505–516. [CrossRef]
33. Sugihara, K.; Kaidzu, S.; Sasaki, M.; Tanito, M. Interventional human ocular safety experiments for 222-nm far-ultraviolet-C lamp irradiation. *Photochem. Photobiol.* 2024, *early view*. [CrossRef]
34. Kolozsvári, L.; Nógrádi, A.; Hopp, B.; Bor, Z. UV Absorbance of the Human Cornea in the 240- to 400-nm Range. *Investig. Ophthalmol. Vis. Sci.* **2002**, *43*, 2165–2168.
35. Schneider, C.A.; Rasband, W.S.; Eliceiri, K.W. NIH Image to ImageJ: 25 years of image analysis. *Nat. Methods* **2012**, *9*, 671–675. [CrossRef]
36. De Vos, K. *Cell Counter*; University of Sheffield, Academic Neurology: Sheffield, UK, 2017.
37. Gierke, A.-M.; Hessling, M. Investigation on Potential ESKAPE Surrogates for 222 and 254 nm Irradiation Experiments. *Front. Microbiol.* **2022**, *13*, 942708. [CrossRef]
38. R Core Team. *R: A Language and Environment for Statistical Computing*; R Foundation for Statistical Computing: Vienna, Austria, 2023.
39. Kim, H.-Y. Statistical notes for clinical researchers: Sample size calculation 1. comparison of two independent sample means. *Restor. Dent. Endod.* **2016**, *41*, 74–78. [CrossRef] [PubMed]
40. Buonanno, M.; Randers-Pehrson, G.; Bigelow, A.W.; Trivedi, S.; Lowy, F.D.; Spotnitz, H.M.; Hammer, S.M.; Brenner, D.J. 207-nm UV light—A promising tool for safe low-cost reduction of surgical site infections. I: In vitro studies. *PLoS ONE* **2013**, *8*, e76968. [CrossRef]
41. Huang, J.-R.; Yang, T.-W.; Hsiao, Y.-I.; Fan, H.-M.; Kuo, H.-Y.; Hung, K.-H.; Chen, P.-Y.; Tan, C.-T.; Shao, P.-L. Far-UVC light (222 nm) efficiently inactivates clinically significant antibiotic-resistant bacteria on diverse material surfaces. *Microbiol. Spectr.* **2024**, *12*, e0425123. [CrossRef] [PubMed]

medicina

MDPI

Review

Enhancing Ophthalmic Diagnosis and Treatment with Artificial Intelligence

David B. Olawade [1,2,3,4,*], Kusal Weerasinghe [2], Mathugamage Don Dasun Eranga Mathugamage [5], Aderonke Odetayo [6], Nicholas Aderinto [7], Jennifer Teke [2,8] and Stergios Boussios [2,8,9,10,11,12]

1 Department of Allied and Public Health, School of Health, Sport and Bioscience, University of East London, London E16 2RD, UK
2 Department of Research and Innovation, Medway NHS Foundation Trust, Gillingham ME7 5NY, UK; kusal.weerasinghe@nhs.net (K.W.); j_teke@nhs.net (J.T.); stergiosboussios@gmail.com (S.B.)
3 Department of Public Health, York St John University, London YO31 7EX, UK
4 School of Health and Care Management, Arden University, Arden House, Middlemarch Park, Coventry CV3 4FJ, UK
5 National Eye Hospital, Colombo 01000, Sri Lanka; dasun1000@gmail.com
6 School of Nursing, Tung Wah College, Hong Kong SAR, China; ronkeodetayo@gmail.com
7 Department of Medicine and Surgery, Ladoke Akintola University of Technology, Ogbomoso 210214, Nigeria; nicholasoluwaseyi6@gmail.com
8 Faculty of Medicine, Health and Social Care, Canterbury Christ Church University, Canterbury CT1 1QU, UK
9 School of Cancer & Pharmaceutical Sciences, King's College London, Strand, London WC2R 2LS, UK
10 Kent Medway Medical School, University of Kent, Canterbury CT2 7NZ, UK
11 Department of Medical Oncology, Medway NHS Foundation Trust, Gillingham ME7 5NK, UK
12 AELIA Organization, 57001 Thessaloniki, Greece
* Correspondence: d.olawade@uel.ac.uk

Abstract: The integration of artificial intelligence (AI) in ophthalmology is transforming the field, offering new opportunities to enhance diagnostic accuracy, personalize treatment plans, and improve service delivery. This review provides a comprehensive overview of the current applications and future potential of AI in ophthalmology. AI algorithms, particularly those utilizing machine learning (ML) and deep learning (DL), have demonstrated remarkable success in diagnosing conditions such as diabetic retinopathy (DR), age-related macular degeneration, and glaucoma with precision comparable to, or exceeding, human experts. Furthermore, AI is being utilized to develop personalized treatment plans by analyzing large datasets to predict individual responses to therapies, thus optimizing patient outcomes and reducing healthcare costs. In surgical applications, AI-driven tools are enhancing the precision of procedures like cataract surgery, contributing to better recovery times and reduced complications. Additionally, AI-powered teleophthalmology services are expanding access to eye care in underserved and remote areas, addressing global disparities in healthcare availability. Despite these advancements, challenges remain, particularly concerning data privacy, security, and algorithmic bias. Ensuring robust data governance and ethical practices is crucial for the continued success of AI integration in ophthalmology. In conclusion, future research should focus on developing sophisticated AI models capable of handling multimodal data, including genetic information and patient histories, to provide deeper insights into disease mechanisms and treatment responses. Also, collaborative efforts among governments, non-governmental organizations (NGOs), and technology companies are essential to deploy AI solutions effectively, especially in low-resource settings.

Keywords: artificial intelligence; ophthalmology; machine learning; diabetic retinopathy; age-related macular degeneration; glaucoma

1. Introduction

Ophthalmology, the branch of medicine dedicated to studying and treating disorders and diseases of the eye and visual system, stands at the forefront of medical innovation. Over the past few decades, technological advancements have significantly transformed the field, enhancing diagnostic accuracy, therapeutic outcomes, and overall patient care [1–3]. One of the most impactful technological advancements in recent years is artificial intelligence (AI), which encompasses both machine learning (ML) and deep learning (DL). AI involves the simulation of human intelligence processes by machines, particularly computer systems. These processes include learning (the acquisition of information and rules for using the information), reasoning (using rules to reach approximate or definite conclusions), and self-correction [4,5]. ML, a subset of AI, enables systems to learn and improve from experience without being explicitly programmed [6]. DL, a further subset of ML, utilizes neural networks with multiple layers to analyze various factors of data [7]. In ophthalmology, AI technologies have shown significant promise in transforming traditional practices. This transformation is driven by the field's heavy reliance on imaging and diagnostic data, which are well suited for AI applications [4,8]. The ability of AI to process and analyze vast amounts of data rapidly and accurately positions it as a revolutionary tool in eye care. For example, a deep learning algorithm has been successfully used to analyze retinal images from a fundus camera to detect early signs of diabetic retinopathy in clinical settings, while machine learning models applied to OCT images have identified subtle retinal changes in patients with AMD [9,10]. These AI applications are highly dependent on the quality and consistency of imaging devices, such as fundus cameras and OCT devices, though they are increasingly integrated with surgical systems like phaco machines to enhance procedural safety [9,11].

One of the most profound impacts of AI in ophthalmology is in the realm of diagnostics. AI systems, particularly those leveraging DL techniques such as convolutional neural networks (CNNs), are adept at recognizing complex patterns in imaging data, which is crucial for diagnosing various eye conditions [7,12]. Diabetic retinopathy (DR) is a significant cause of blindness among working-age adults worldwide [13]. Traditional diagnostic methods rely on the manual examination of retinal images, which can be time-consuming and subject to human error. AI algorithms, however, have demonstrated the ability to detect DR with high sensitivity and specificity [9,10]. Notably, the study by Gulshan et al. highlighted an AI system capable of identifying DR in retinal images with performance comparable to that of experienced ophthalmologists [10]. Such advancements ensure that patients at risk of vision loss are identified and treated promptly, thus preventing disease progression. Age-related macular degeneration (AMD) is another major cause of vision loss, particularly among the elderly. Early detection and monitoring are critical in managing AMD, and AI has proven to be a valuable tool in this regard [11]. AI models have been developed to analyze optical coherence tomography (OCT) images, differentiating between normal and pathological features with remarkable accuracy. For instance, research has shown that AI algorithms can classify AMD stages from OCT scans, providing crucial support for early intervention and personalized treatment strategies [11,14].

Glaucoma, often referred to as the "silent thief of sight", is characterized by optic nerve damage and is a leading cause of irreversible blindness [15,16]. Early detection and continuous monitoring are essential for managing glaucoma. AI applications, particularly those involving the automated analysis of OCT images and visual field tests, have shown significant promise [17,18]. In the context of glaucoma, while traditional trend analysis of visual field parameters relies on observing longitudinal changes, AI-based prediction leverages complex patterns from multimodal data to forecast progression with greater sensitivity and specificity [17]. These AI tools assist ophthalmologists in detecting early signs of glaucoma and tracking disease progression, facilitating timely and effective interventions.

In addition to its diagnostic capabilities, AI is revolutionizing the treatment and management of ophthalmic diseases. Personalized medicine, which tailors treatment plans to individual patient profiles, is significantly enhanced by AI's ability to analyze extensive datasets and predict treatment outcomes [19,20]. AI can analyze data from diverse sources, including patient demographics, medical history, genetic information, and imaging data, to develop personalized treatment plans [19]. In the context of ophthalmology, this capability is particularly valuable. For example, AI-driven models can predict which patients with DR are likely to respond to specific treatments, enabling more targeted and effective interventions [9]. Moreover, advancements in AI-guided surgical tools—such as those that stabilize the anterior chamber during cataract surgery or automate instrument calibration in vitreoretinal procedures—have already been incorporated into routine practice, subtly enhancing the ease and safety of surgical procedures [21].

AI is not only transforming clinical practice but also enhancing service delivery in ophthalmology. By automating routine tasks and optimizing workflows, AI can significantly improve efficiency and patient care [21,22]. AI-powered screening programs are being implemented to improve access to eye care [23,24], especially in remote and underserved areas [25]. Mobile applications and teleophthalmology services utilize AI to screen for common eye diseases, such as DR and glaucoma [26,27], facilitating early detection and timely referral to specialists. These programs are particularly beneficial in addressing disparities in eye care access, ensuring that more people receive the necessary care. In clinical settings, AI can streamline workflows by automating routine tasks, such as image analysis and patient triage [9,22]. This not only enhances efficiency but also allows ophthalmologists to focus on more complex cases, thereby improving the overall quality of care. AI-driven systems can prioritize patients based on the severity of their conditions, ensuring that those in urgent need receive prompt attention [20].

The rationale for this study is grounded in the transformative potential of AI to revolutionize ophthalmic practices. Traditional diagnostic methods in ophthalmology, often reliant on subjective interpretation and manual analysis, face limitations in terms of efficiency and accuracy [9]. With the rising prevalence of eye diseases like DR, AMD, and glaucoma, there is an urgent need for advanced diagnostic and treatment tools. AI-powered screening programs and teleophthalmology services present significant opportunities to address the global burden of eye diseases [26].

The objectives of this study are multifaceted, aiming to provide a comprehensive overview of AI applications in ophthalmology, assess the benefits and challenges of integrating AI into clinical practice, and explore future directions for AI-driven advancements in the field. The main objective of this narrative review is to systematically evaluate the current landscape of AI technologies in ophthalmology by addressing the following research questions: (1) What are the specific AI tools and techniques currently employed in ophthalmic diagnosis, treatment, and service delivery? (2) What benefits and challenges are associated with their integration into clinical practice? (3) What future trends and directions can be anticipated for AI-driven innovations in this field?

The novelty of this review lies in its holistic approach, examining not only individual AI tools and techniques but also their integration across various data modalities to offer more comprehensive insights into eye diseases and treatments. Furthermore, the study emphasizes the role of AI in personalizing treatment plans, improving service delivery through teleophthalmology, and addressing ethical and practical challenges associated with AI implementation. By highlighting emerging trends and potential advancements, this study aims to provide a forward-looking perspective that can inform both clinical practice and future research, ultimately contributing to the responsible and effective use of AI in ophthalmology. Figure 1 below shows various applications of AI in ophthalmology domains.

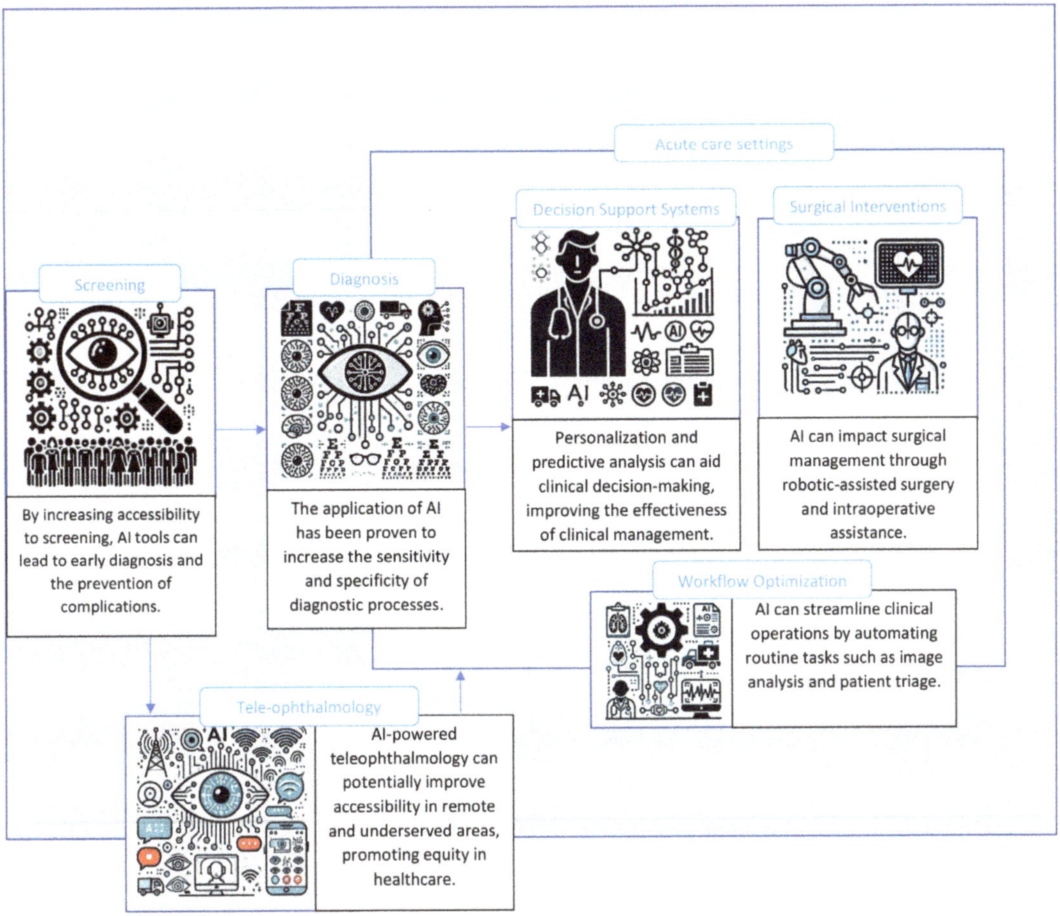

Figure 1. AI applications in various ophthalmology domains.

2. Methodology

This narrative review employs a comprehensive literature review methodology to gather, analyze, and synthesize existing research on the applications of AI in ophthalmology. The methodology includes several key steps: defining the research scope, selecting relevant databases, establishing inclusion and exclusion criteria, conducting a systematic search, and analyzing and synthesizing the collected data.

2.1. Database Selection and Search Strategy

Relevant peer-reviewed articles, conference papers, and review articles were identified using multiple scientific databases, including PubMed, Google Scholar, IEEE Xplore, and ScienceDirect. The search strategy involved the use of keywords and phrases such as "AI in ophthalmology", "machine learning in eye care", "deep learning in ophthalmic diagnosis", "AI in diabetic retinopathy", "AI in glaucoma detection", "teleophthalmology", and "AI in personalized medicine for eye diseases". Boolean operators (AND, OR) were employed to refine and expand the search to capture a comprehensive set of relevant studies.

2.2. Inclusion and Exclusion Criteria

To ensure the relevance and quality of the reviewed literature, specific inclusion and exclusion criteria were established. The included studies were those that met the following criteria:

- Focus on the application of AI in ophthalmology.
- Are peer-reviewed and published within the last ten years (2013–2023) to ensure contemporary relevance.
- Provide empirical data, case studies, systematic reviews, or meta-analyses on the use of AI in diagnosing, treating, or managing eye diseases.
- Discuss ethical, practical, or future-oriented aspects of AI in ophthalmology.

Studies were excluded if they met the following criteria:

- Do not specifically address AI applications in ophthalmology.
- Are opinion pieces, editorials, or anecdotal reports without empirical data.
- Are published in non-English languages, due to language constraints.

2.3. Systematic Search and Data Extraction

A systematic search of the selected databases was conducted using predefined keywords and criteria. Titles and abstracts of the retrieved articles were screened for relevance, and full-text versions of potentially relevant articles were obtained for detailed review. A data extraction form was used to systematically collect information from each included study, including study objectives, methods, AI techniques used, findings, benefits, challenges, and future recommendations.

2.4. Data Analysis and Synthesis

The extracted data were analyzed using qualitative synthesis methods. The studies were categorized based on their primary focus: diagnostic applications, therapeutic applications, service delivery improvements, and ethical considerations. Within each category, thematic analysis was conducted to identify common themes, trends, and gaps in the literature. The findings were then synthesized to provide a comprehensive overview of the current state of AI in ophthalmology, highlighting key advancements, benefits, challenges, and future directions.

3. AI in Ophthalmic Diagnosis

Table 1 below highlights the diverse applications of AI in ophthalmic diagnosis, emphasizing the technology, key systems, accuracy, clinical applications, advantages, and challenges for various eye conditions. AI algorithms for glaucoma predict disease progression and assist in timely intervention [28]. ML models streamline cataract diagnosis by automating assessment and grading from slit-lamp images [29,30]. DL models for retinal vein occlusion (RVO) enhance diagnostic precision, reducing manual analysis [31,32]. AI integration of genetic data with imaging for retinitis pigmentosa offers comprehensive disease insights [33,34]. AI-powered corneal topography for keratoconus ensures early detection and better treatment outcomes [35]. AI applications in ocular surface diseases improve patient management and reduce workload [36]. For uveitis, AI combines imaging and clinical data for early detection and tailored treatment plans [37,38]. Despite these advancements, challenges like data privacy, algorithmic bias, workflow integration, and model generalizability persist across applications [39].

Table 1. AI in ophthalmic diagnosis.

Condition	AI Technology	Clinical Application	Advantages	Challenges
DR	CNNs	Automated screening from retinal images	High diagnostic accuracy, reduced screening time	Data privacy, algorithmic bias, integration with EHR
AMD	DL	Classification of AMD stages from OCT images	Early detection, improved patient outcomes	Training in diverse datasets, regulatory compliance
Glaucoma	AI algorithms for OCT and visual field analysis	Early diagnosis and monitoring through automated analysis of OCT and visual fields	Timely intervention, reduced vision loss	Data accuracy, handling large datasets
Cataract	ML models	Diagnosis and grading of cataracts from slit-lamp images	Automated assessment, standardized grading	Integration into clinical workflows, user training
RVO	DL models	Detection and classification of RVO from OCT images	Accurate diagnosis, reduced need for manual analysis	Ensuring model generalizability, data sharing
Retinitis Pigmentosa	Genetic data integration with imaging AI	Combined genetic and imaging analysis for early diagnosis	Comprehensive insights into disease mechanisms	Ethical considerations, data privacy
Keratoconus	AI for corneal topography	Early detection from corneal topography images	Early intervention, improved treatment outcomes	Ensuring algorithm fairness, handling complex data
Ocular Surface Diseases	ML and image analysis	Detection and monitoring of ocular surface conditions from slit-lamp and tear film images	Improved patient management, reduced workload	Data integration, maintaining data privacy
Uveitis	AI for imaging and clinical data	Diagnosis and monitoring from multimodal imaging and clinical data	Early detection, tailored treatment plans	Data complexity, ensuring unbiased algorithms

Abbreviations—AI: artificial intelligence; DR: diabetic retinopathy; CNNs: convolutional neural networks; EHR: electronic health records; AMD: age-related macular degeneration; DL: deep learning; OCT: optical coherence tomography; ML: machine learning; and RVO: retinal vein occlusion.

3.1. Diabetic Retinopathy

DR is a leading cause of blindness worldwide, primarily affecting individuals with diabetes [40,41]. It is characterized by damage to the blood vessels of the retina, which can lead to vision impairment and, ultimately, blindness if left untreated. Early detection and timely intervention are crucial to preventing vision loss [40]. However, traditional methods for diagnosing DR rely on manual examination of retinal images by ophthalmologists, which can be time-consuming and prone to variability [33,40].

AI algorithms, especially CNNs, have demonstrated remarkable accuracy in detecting DR from retinal images. CNNs are well suited for image analysis tasks due to their ability to automatically learn and extract features from raw image data, enabling them to identify patterns and anomalies indicative of DR [42,43]. Numerous studies have shown that AI can achieve sensitivity and specificity comparable to, or even surpass, human experts in detecting DR [10,42–45]. One of the most notable AI systems for DR detection is the EyeArt AI system. EyeArt has been extensively validated in clinical settings and has shown over 90% sensitivity in detecting referable DR, which refers to cases that require further evaluation by an ophthalmologist [42,46]. A pivotal study involving EyeArt demonstrated its ability to accurately identify DR in a diverse patient population, highlighting its potential as a reliable screening tool [46]. However, it is important to note that according to WHO criteria for a valid screening program, a system must achieve at least ≥80% sensitivity and ≥95% specificity; while EyeArt demonstrates sensitivity over 90%, its specificity has been reported in some studies to fall below the 95% threshold [42,46]. The system's high sensitivity ensures that most cases of referable DR are detected, thereby reducing the risk of missed diagnoses and facilitating early intervention.

Another prominent AI model is the system developed by Google Health, which utilizes DL techniques to analyze retinal photographs [10,12]. This AI model has been trained on a large dataset of retinal images labeled by expert ophthalmologists. In a recent study, the Google Health model achieved sensitivity and specificity rates comparable to those of board-certified ophthalmologists [10,47]. The model's ability to accurately identify both referable and non-referable DR underscores its potential to enhance screening programs and improve access to eye care, particularly in resource-limited settings.

Comparative studies have further underscored the efficacy of AI in DR detection. For example, a study comparing the performance of several AI models, including EyeArt and Google Health's system, found that these AI tools consistently outperformed traditional manual grading by ophthalmologists in terms of both speed and accuracy [12,42,45]. These findings suggest that AI can serve as a valuable adjunct to human expertise, enabling more efficient and reliable screening processes. In real-world applications, AI systems for DR detection have been deployed in various settings, from urban hospitals to rural clinics [12,46]. The scalability and accessibility of AI technologies make them particularly advantageous for large-scale screening programs. For instance, in India, where the prevalence of diabetes is high and access to specialized eye care is limited, AI-based screening initiatives have been implemented to identify patients at risk of DR [47]. These programs leverage AI to analyze retinal images captured by mobile screening units, providing immediate feedback and referral recommendations [10,43]. The integration of AI in such programs has demonstrated significant improvements in screening coverage and diagnostic accuracy, ultimately contributing to better patient outcomes.

3.2. *Age-Related Macular Degeneration*

AMD is a leading cause of vision loss, particularly among older adults. It affects the macula, the part of the retina responsible for central vision, leading to progressive vision impairment and, in severe cases, blindness [48]. Early and accurate diagnosis is crucial for managing AMD and preventing severe visual deterioration. Traditional diagnostic methods include clinical examination and imaging techniques, such as OCT [49,50]. However, these methods can be time-consuming and require significant expertise.

AI systems have been developed to classify AMD stages from OCT images with remarkable accuracy. These systems utilize DL algorithms, such as CNNs, to analyze the intricate details of retinal images and distinguish between normal and pathological features [45,51]. By processing large volumes of data, AI models can learn to identify the subtle signs of early AMD, intermediate stages, and advanced forms of the disease, including both dry and wet AMD [11,52]. In clinical validation studies, the DL system achieved diagnostic accuracy comparable to that of experienced retinal specialists [12,53]. This level of precision highlights the potential of AI to assist in early detection and monitoring, enabling timely interventions that can slow disease progression and preserve vision.

The integration of AI into AMD diagnosis provides substantial support to ophthalmologists. AI models can rapidly analyze OCT scans and flag images that exhibit signs of AMD, prioritizing patients who need immediate attention [44,50]. This triage capability reduces the diagnostic burden on ophthalmologists, allowing them to focus on patients with more complex cases [11,52]. For instance, studies have shown that AI-driven analysis of OCT images can significantly decrease the time required for initial screenings, freeing up resources and improving the efficiency of eye care services [12,54]. Additionally, AI systems can provide continuous monitoring for patients with AMD. By comparing sequential OCT images, AI can detect subtle changes that may indicate disease progression or response to treatment [52,55].

In real-world clinical settings, AI systems for AMD detection and classification have shown promising results. For example, the Moorfields–DeepMind collaboration developed an AI system capable of diagnosing a wide range of retinal diseases, including AMD, from OCT scans [12,56]. The system was tested in clinical practice and demonstrated high accuracy, often exceeding that of human experts. This collaboration highlighted the potential for AI to be integrated into routine clinical workflows, providing reliable and scalable diagnostic support. Another significant application is the use of AI in large-scale screening programs. In regions with limited access to specialized eye care, AI-powered screening tools can facilitate early detection of AMD and other retinal diseases [11,57]. Mobile screening units equipped with OCT devices and AI analysis capabilities can reach underserved populations, providing immediate feedback and referral recommendations [58,59]. These programs have shown success in identifying individuals at risk and ensuring they receive timely and appropriate care.

3.3. *Glaucoma*

Glaucoma is a group of eye conditions characterized by damage to the optic nerve, often associated with elevated intraocular pressure [16,60]. It is one of the leading causes of irreversible blindness worldwide [60,61]. Early detection and continuous monitoring are crucial to prevent significant vision loss, as the damage caused by glaucoma is typically asymptomatic in the early stages. AI applications have shown great promise in improving the diagnosis and management of glaucoma through the automated analysis of OCT images and visual field tests [62,63]. Studies have demonstrated that AI systems can reliably identify glaucomatous changes in the optic nerve head and retinal nerve fiber layer [28,64]. For instance, an AI model developed by researchers at Moorfields Eye Hospital and DeepMind was trained on a large dataset of OCT images and demonstrated performance comparable to that of expert ophthalmologists in diagnosing glaucoma [12,55]. This model could detect structural abnormalities associated with glaucoma and provide diagnostic suggestions with high sensitivity and specificity. By automating the detection of glaucoma-related changes, AI systems can assist ophthalmologists in identifying patients at risk of glaucoma earlier than conventional methods [28,63].

Visual field testing is another essential component in diagnosing and monitoring glaucoma. It measures a patient's peripheral vision and helps identify functional loss caused by optic nerve damage [65,66]. Traditional visual field tests often rely on trend analysis—using statistical methods such as linear regression to evaluate changes in visual field parameters over time—which can be subjective and influenced by patient performance, leading to variability in results. In contrast, AI-based prediction leverages complex pattern recognition from the entire dataset, including nonlinear trends, to forecast disease progression with greater sensitivity and specificity [63,67]. ML algorithms can analyze patterns in visual field data to detect early glaucomatous changes and predict disease progression [68]. One significant study by Medeiros et al. demonstrated that an AI algorithm could predict the future progression of visual field loss in glaucoma patients with high accuracy [69]. The algorithm analyzed longitudinal visual field data, identifying patterns that indicated the likelihood of disease progression. This predictive capability allows for more proactive management of glaucoma, enabling timely interventions to prevent further vision loss.

AI tools for glaucoma diagnosis and monitoring have been validated in clinical settings, showing substantial benefits in improving patient care [12,17]. For example, AI-powered platforms that integrate OCT analysis and visual field data have been implemented in ophthalmology clinics to assist clinicians in making more informed decisions [69]. These platforms provide a comprehensive assessment of glaucoma, combining structural and functional data to offer a holistic view of the disease [18,61]. In community screening programs, AI systems have been used to identify individuals at risk of glaucoma, particularly in underserved areas where access to specialist eye care is limited [25,70]. This approach has been shown to increase the detection rates of glaucoma and facilitate earlier treatment.

4. AI in Treatment and Management

4.1. Personalized Treatment Plans

AI models, particularly those based on ML and DL techniques, have shown remarkable ability in predicting disease progression and treatment outcomes. By analyzing diverse data sources such as patient demographics, genetic information, imaging data, and treatment histories, AI can generate precise predictions tailored to individual patients [22,71]. Researchers have developed models that analyze retinal images and other relevant data to forecast the likelihood of disease worsening [9,10,45]. These predictions enable ophthalmologists to tailor treatment plans according to the specific needs of each patient, such as adjusting the frequency of monitoring visits or the type of interventions.

Similarly, in AMD management, AI-driven models can analyze OCT images along with clinical data to predict how patients will respond to various treatments, such as anti-vascular endothelial growth factor (anti-VEGF) injections [11,51,72]. Studies have shown that AI can identify patients who are likely to benefit from specific therapies and those who may require alternative treatment strategies [1,22,57]. This capability allows for more targeted and effective interventions, improving patient outcomes and reducing unnecessary treatments.

AI's ability to analyze complex datasets and recognize patterns that may not be apparent to human clinicians plays a crucial role in optimizing therapeutic strategies. By continuously learning from new data, AI models can refine their predictions and recommendations, ensuring that treatment plans remain up to date with the latest clinical insights and patient responses [12,22,71]. AI models can predict which patients are at higher risk of rapid disease progression and require more aggressive treatment, such as early surgical intervention, versus those who can be managed with less intensive therapies [58,73]. This individualized approach helps in allocating resources more efficiently and improving the quality of care.

The application of AI in personalizing treatment plans has shown promising results in improving patient outcomes and reducing treatment costs. By accurately predicting disease progression and tailoring interventions, AI helps in achieving better clinical outcomes with fewer complications [45]. Early and precise interventions can prevent the progression of eye diseases, reducing the need for more extensive and costly treatments later on. In addition to clinical benefits, AI-driven personalized treatment plans can lead to significant cost savings for healthcare systems [45,74]. By optimizing the use of resources and minimizing unnecessary treatments, AI contributes to more efficient healthcare delivery. For instance, AI models can help determine the optimal frequency of anti-VEGF injections for AMD patients, reducing the number of injections needed while maintaining therapeutic efficacy [52,72]. This not only lowers treatment costs but also improves patient compliance and satisfaction.

4.2. Surgical Applications

AI is transforming ophthalmic surgery by enhancing precision, reducing complications, and improving patient outcomes through robotic-assisted surgery and AI-guided instruments [75–77]. These advanced technologies provide real-time feedback, assist in making accurate incisions, and optimize various surgical procedures, such as cataract surgery [77,78]. Traditional cataract surgery involves manually removing the cloudy lens and replacing it with an artificial lens. This procedure requires steady hands and precise movements, as even minor deviations can lead to complications [78]. Robotic-assisted surgery is revolutionizing the field of ophthalmology by providing surgeons with enhanced control and precision. AI-powered robotic systems can assist in performing intricate surgical tasks that require a high degree of accuracy [79,80]. One of the key advantages of robotic-assisted surgery is its ability to reduce human error [76,81]. Robotic systems equipped with AI algorithms can stabilize the surgical instruments and perform precise maneuvers, minimizing the risk of errors. In addition, modern phaco devices are designed to automatically regulate fluidics to maintain a stable anterior chamber during cataract surgery, which reduces intraoperative fluctuations and protects the corneal endothelium. Furthermore, features such as real-time intraoperative imaging overlays and automated fluid management systems have been seamlessly integrated into everyday surgical practice, providing subtle yet significant improvements that enhance surgical safety and ease without drawing undue attention from the surgeon.

AI-guided instruments are another significant innovation in ophthalmic surgery. For example, in retinal surgery, AI-guided instruments can assist surgeons in making precise incisions and accurately positioning implants [75,82]. AI algorithms can analyze intraoperative data, such as imaging and sensor information, to provide surgeons with critical insights [77,80]. This real-time analysis helps in identifying optimal incision sites, avoiding critical structures, and ensuring proper alignment of surgical instruments.

Cataract surgery is one of the most common ophthalmic procedures, and AI is playing a crucial role in enhancing its precision and outcomes. AI-powered robotic systems can assist in various stages of cataract surgery, from preoperative planning to intraoperative execution [77,82]. Preoperative planning involves creating a detailed map of the patient's eye to guide the surgical procedure [75]. AI algorithms can analyze diagnostic images and generate a precise surgical plan, including the optimal size and location of the incisions and the appropriate power and position of the intraocular lens [83,84]. This personalized approach ensures that the surgery is tailored to the individual patient's anatomy, leading to better visual outcomes. During the surgery, AI-guided instruments provide real-time feedback to the surgeon, helping them make accurate incisions and perform delicate maneuvers [85]. For instance, femtosecond laser-assisted cataract surgery utilizes AI to control the laser, making precise corneal incisions and fragmenting the cataract with high accuracy [82,85]. This technology reduces the risk of complications, such as capsular tears and corneal astigmatism, and shortens the recovery time for patients.

AI-assisted ophthalmic surgery offers several benefits in terms of reducing complications and improving recovery times. By enhancing surgical precision and minimizing human error, AI technologies help lower the incidence of postoperative complications [81,84]. Moreover, AI can contribute to faster recovery times by ensuring that surgical procedures are performed with minimal trauma to the surrounding tissues [75]. Precise incisions and optimized surgical techniques reduce inflammation and promote quicker healing [85]. Patients undergoing AI-assisted cataract surgery often experience faster visual recovery and improved overall satisfaction.

5. AI in Ophthalmology Service Delivery

AI is revolutionizing service delivery in ophthalmology by automating routine tasks, optimizing workflows, and enhancing efficiency in patient care [86]. These advancements are particularly impactful in screening programs, where AI-powered solutions improve access to eye care, especially in remote and underserved areas [8,87]. Table 2 below outlines various AI applications in ophthalmology service delivery, detailing the technologies, key systems, clinical applications, advantages, and challenges associated with each area, including screening programs, teleophthalmology, workflow optimization, patient monitoring, decision support systems, resource allocation, and patient engagement.

Table 2. AI in ophthalmology service delivery.

Service Area	AI Technology	Key Systems/ Programs	Clinical Application	Advantages	Challenges
Screening Programs	AI-powered screening tools	EyeArt, IDx-DR, mobile AI apps	Early detection of eye diseases, such as DR and glaucoma	Increased access, early detection, reduced workload	Data privacy, ensuring accuracy in diverse settings
Teleophthalmology	AI in telemedicine platforms	Retina-AI, telehealth initiatives	Remote diagnosis and monitoring of eye conditions	Access to care in remote areas, timely referrals	Technology access, maintaining data security
Workflow Optimization	AI for task automation	AI-driven triage and scheduling	Automating image analysis, patient triage, and scheduling	Improved efficiency, allowing for focus on complex cases	Interoperability with existing systems, user acceptance
Patient Monitoring	AI in wearable devices	Smart contact lenses, AI apps	Continuous monitoring of eye conditions	Real-time data, proactive management	Data management, patient adherence
Decision Support Systems	Clinical decision support AI	IBM Watson, Google Health AI	Assisting in diagnosis and treatment planning	Enhanced decision-making, personalized care	Trust in AI recommendations, integration into workflow
Resource Allocation	AI for resource management	Hospital management AI tools	Optimizing use of medical resources and staff scheduling	Cost savings, improved resource utilization	Implementation costs, training staff
Patient Engagement	AI chatbots and virtual assistants	Chatbots for appointment scheduling, symptom checking	Enhancing patient communication and education	Improved patient satisfaction, reduced administrative burden	Accuracy of AI responses, patient data privacy

Abbreviations—AI: artificial intelligence; DR: diabetic retinopathy.

5.1. Screening Programs

AI-powered screening programs are transforming the landscape of ophthalmic care by enabling large-scale, efficient, and accurate screening processes. These programs utilize advanced algorithms to analyze retinal images and other relevant data, identifying signs of eye diseases with high accuracy [8,87]. The implementation of AI in screening programs offers several benefits, including improved access to care, early detection, and reduced healthcare costs [88,89]. Mobile applications and teleophthalmology services are at the forefront of AI-driven screening programs. These platforms allow for remote screening of eye diseases, making it possible to reach populations that lack access to traditional eye care services [26,90]. AI algorithms integrated into mobile apps can analyze images captured by smartphone cameras or portable retinal imaging devices, providing immediate diagnostic feedback.

Teleophthalmology services extend the reach of AI-powered screening by connecting patients in remote areas with specialists in urban centers [26,91]. Retinal images and other relevant data are transmitted to centralized AI systems for analysis. The results are then reviewed by ophthalmologists who can provide detailed assessments and recommendations [8,90]. This model has been successfully implemented in various regions, significantly reducing the barriers to accessing specialized eye care.

In many parts of the world, there is a shortage of trained ophthalmologists, and patients in rural or underserved areas often face long travel distances to receive care. AI-driven screening tools can bridge this gap by providing accurate and timely diagnoses at the point of care [84,87]. One notable example is the implementation of AI screening programs in India, where DR is a major public health concern [45,47,92]. AI-powered systems have been integrated into primary care settings, allowing healthcare workers to screen patients and refer those with positive findings to specialized eye care centers [22,84,91]. This approach has significantly increased the detection rates of DR and reduced the burden on tertiary care centers.

The automation of routine screening tasks through AI not only improves efficiency but also reduces healthcare costs by reducing the need for unnecessary referrals and follow-up visits [21,71,89]. By accurately identifying patients who need further evaluation, AI systems help ensure that healthcare resources are used more effectively. This targeted approach minimizes the financial burden on both healthcare systems and patients. Furthermore, AI-powered screening programs can integrate with electronic health records (EHR) systems, streamlining the documentation and management of patient data [22,71]. Automated data entry and analysis reduce administrative workloads, allowing healthcare providers to allocate more time to patient care.

The real-world application of AI in ophthalmology service delivery has yielded numerous success stories. For example, the EyePACS program in the United States uses AI to screen for DR in underserved populations [26,93]. This program has successfully screened millions of patients, identifying those at risk and facilitating timely treatment. The AI system used in EyePACS has demonstrated high accuracy, comparable to that of human graders, highlighting the potential of AI to enhance screening programs on a large scale [42]. Another success story comes from the United Kingdom, where the National Health Service (NHS) has implemented AI-powered screening for DR [8,23]. The AI system analyzes retinal images and flags those that require further review by an ophthalmologist. This approach has improved the efficiency of the screening process and ensured that patients with sight-threatening retinopathy receive prompt care.

5.2. *Workflow Optimization*

AI is significantly enhancing workflow optimization in ophthalmology by automating routine tasks, such as image analysis and patient triage [9,84,94]. This not only improves efficiency but also allows ophthalmologists to focus on more complex cases, ultimately enhancing overall service delivery. One of the key areas where AI is making a substantial impact is in the automation of routine tasks. Image analysis, a critical component of ophthalmic diagnostics, can be time-consuming and labor-intensive. AI algorithms, particularly those based on deep learning, can analyze large volumes of imaging data quickly and accurately [4,73].

By automating image analysis, AI significantly reduces the workload of ophthalmologists and technicians [1,84]. This not only speeds up the diagnostic process but also ensures a high level of consistency and accuracy in the interpretation of imaging data. Studies have shown that AI algorithms can match or even exceed the diagnostic accuracy of human experts in detecting various eye conditions [3,12,84,90]. This allows for a more efficient allocation of human resources, enabling clinicians to dedicate their time and expertise to more complex and critical cases.

Patient triage is another area where AI is optimizing clinical workflows. Efficient triage systems are essential for prioritizing patients based on the urgency and severity of their conditions. AI-driven triage systems use advanced algorithms to analyze patient data, including medical histories, symptoms, and imaging results, to determine the urgency of each case [22,71]. This prioritization ensures that patients with severe conditions receive timely care, reducing the risk of complications and improving overall outcomes. AI-based triage systems can also provide decision support to clinicians, offering recommendations on the appropriate course of action for each patient [95].

AI's ability to streamline clinical workflows extends beyond image analysis and triage. By integrating with EHR systems, AI can automate various administrative tasks, such as data entry, documentation, and appointment scheduling [2,21]. This integration enhances the overall efficiency of clinical operations and reduces the administrative burden on healthcare providers. For instance, AI algorithms can extract relevant information from EHRs and populate patient records automatically, ensuring that the data are accurately recorded and readily available for clinical decision-making. Additionally, AI can optimize appointment scheduling by predicting no-show rates and adjusting schedules, accordingly, maximizing the utilization of clinical resources [21].

A notable example of AI optimizing workflow in ophthalmology is its application in glaucoma management. Glaucoma requires regular monitoring of intraocular pressure, visual fields, and optic nerve health [16]. AI-driven platforms can automate the analysis of visual field tests and OCT images, providing consistent and objective assessments [63]. These platforms can detect subtle changes in the optic nerve head and retinal nerve fiber layer, which are critical for early diagnosis and monitoring of glaucoma [17,64]. Moreover, AI systems can integrate data from multiple sources to provide a comprehensive risk assessment for each patient [22,73]. For example, combining IOP measurements, visual field data, and OCT results, AI can predict the risk of glaucoma progression and recommend personalized monitoring and treatment plans. This approach not only enhances the efficiency of clinical workflows but also improves patient outcomes by enabling early and targeted interventions.

6. Challenges and Ethical Considerations

6.1. Data Privacy and Security

The integration of AI in ophthalmology brings significant benefits but also raises critical concerns about data privacy and security. The confidentiality and integrity of patient data must be maintained to ensure trust and compliance with regulatory standards. This section explores the challenges associated with data privacy and security in AI-driven ophthalmology and the measures needed to address these issues. One of the primary concerns in AI-driven ophthalmology is ensuring that patient data remain confidential and secure [96,97]. AI systems often require access to large datasets, including retinal images, medical histories, and demographic information, to train algorithms and improve diagnostic accuracy [21]. The collection, storage, and processing of this sensitive information pose significant privacy risks. To ensure data confidentiality, robust encryption methods must be employed both in transit and at rest [97]. This means that data should be encrypted when they are being transmitted over networks and when they are stored in databases. Encryption ensures that unauthorized parties cannot access or tamper with the data, thereby maintaining its integrity [98]. Additionally, access controls must be strictly enforced to ensure that only authorized personnel can access sensitive patient data. This includes implementing multi-factor authentication (MFA) and role-based access control (RBAC) to limit access based on the user's role and necessity. Regular audits and monitoring of access logs are also essential to detect and respond to unauthorized access attempts promptly [99].

Robust data governance frameworks are crucial for protecting sensitive information and ensuring compliance with regulatory standards, such as the General Data Protection Regulation (GDPR) in Europe, the Health Insurance Portability and Accountability Act (HIPAA) in the United States, and other national data protection laws [100,101]. These frameworks provide guidelines and policies for data collection, storage, processing, and sharing, ensuring that patient data are handled ethically and legally. Key components of an effective data governance framework include data minimization, data anonymization, data retention policies, consent management, and transparency and accountability [102,103]. Data minimization involves collecting only the data necessary for specific AI applications to reduce the risk of exposure [104]. Data anonymization involves removing or masking personally identifiable information (PII) to protect patient privacy while allowing for data analysis [105,106]. Data retention policies establish clear guidelines on how long data should be retained and ensure their secure disposal when no longer needed [107]. Consent management ensures that patients provide informed consent for the use of their data, with clear explanations of how it will be used and the benefits and risks involved [108].

Compliance with regulatory standards is essential for maintaining trust and ensuring that AI applications in ophthalmology adhere to legal and ethical guidelines. Regulations such as GDPR and HIPAA set stringent requirements for data protection, including the rights of individuals to access, correct, and delete their data, and the obligation of organizations to report data breaches promptly [100,101]. To comply with these standards, organizations must implement comprehensive data protection measures. These measures include conducting Data Protection Impact Assessments (DPIAs) to identify and mitigate potential privacy risks associated with AI applications; establishing breach notification procedures to detect, report, and respond to data breaches in a timely manner [109]; ensuring staff training and awareness in data protection principles and practices; and managing vendors to ensure that third-party vendors and partners comply with data protection standards and contractual obligations to safeguard patient data [110].

6.2. Bias and Fairness

AI algorithms, despite their transformative potential in ophthalmology, can inadvertently introduce biases that lead to disparities in patient care [111]. The primary sources of bias in AI systems include the training data, algorithm design, and operational implementation. Training data bias occurs when the datasets used are not representative of the broader population, such as a retinal image dataset dominated by images from a single demographic group, which may result in algorithms that perform inadequately on other demographic groups [111,112]. Algorithm design bias can stem from developer decisions regarding feature selection, model architecture, and hyperparameter tuning. Operational bias arises during the deployment and use of AI systems, where the interaction with clinical workflows and the interpretation of AI outputs by healthcare providers may introduce unintended biases [113].

To ensure fairness and generalizability in AI models, it is imperative to develop and validate these models using diverse and representative datasets. In ophthalmology, this means including retinal images from patients with diverse skin tones, ages, and underlying health conditions [114]. Bias detection and mitigation techniques should be employed during the training process to identify and address biases [112,114]. Fairness metrics can be used to assess the performance of AI models across different subgroups, and techniques such as reweighting or resampling data, adversarial debiasing methods, and incorporating fairness constraints in training can help reduce bias [112,115].

Robust validation of AI models on independent and diverse datasets not used during training is essential to ensure these models generalize well to new, unseen data. This involves using cross-validation techniques and conducting external validation studies to test the model's performance across various population groups [116]. Continuous monitoring and updating of AI systems are necessary to maintain their fairness and reliability over time [117]. This ongoing process helps to identify new biases as they emerge and adjust the models accordingly.

6.3. Integration into Clinical Practice

Integrating AI into existing clinical workflows in ophthalmology poses several challenges, particularly concerning interoperability and user acceptance. For AI tools to be effectively utilized, they must seamlessly integrate with the current healthcare infrastructure, including EHRs and other clinical systems [22,71]. This requires robust interoperability standards to ensure that AI systems can communicate and exchange data with these existing platforms without disruption.

One of the primary hurdles in integrating AI into clinical practice is ensuring that healthcare professionals are adequately trained to use these tools. This involves not only technical training but also educating clinicians on the benefits and limitations of AI systems [71,74,118,119]. By providing comprehensive training programs, healthcare organizations can help clinicians become proficient in using AI tools, thereby improving user acceptance and confidence in these technologies [71,118]. Addressing concerns about job displacement is also critical. AI should be positioned as a tool that enhances the capabilities of healthcare professionals rather than replacing them [71]. By automating routine tasks and providing decision support, AI can free up clinicians to focus on more complex and patient-centric activities, ultimately improving patient care.

Successful implementation of AI in ophthalmology requires collaborative efforts between technologists and clinicians [84]. This collaboration is essential for designing AI solutions that are both user-friendly and clinically relevant. Clinicians can provide valuable insights into the practical challenges and needs of clinical practice, while technologists can offer expertise in developing sophisticated AI algorithms and systems [84,120]. Together, they can create AI tools that fit seamlessly into clinical workflows and address real-world clinical problems. For example, incorporating feedback from ophthalmologists during the development phase can lead to the creation of AI tools that are intuitive and tailored to the specific needs of eye care.

Furthermore, it is important to engage in continuous dialogue with all stakeholders, including patients, to ensure that AI systems meet their needs and expectations [22,121,122]. Patient education and transparency about how AI is used in their care can enhance trust and acceptance [123]. By fostering a culture of collaboration and open communication, healthcare organizations can facilitate the integration of AI into clinical practice, ensuring that these technologies are embraced and effectively utilized to enhance patient outcomes.

7. Future Directions

7.1. Enhanced AI Models

The future of AI in ophthalmology lies in the development of more sophisticated models capable of handling multimodal data, which include not only imaging data but also genetic information, patient histories, and other relevant clinical data. Such comprehensive models have the potential to revolutionize our understanding of disease mechanisms and enhance the precision of treatment responses. One promising direction for future research is the integration of genetic data with traditional imaging and clinical data [124]. By combining these diverse data types, AI models can offer a more holistic view of a patient's health, potentially identifying genetic predispositions to certain eye diseases and predicting how these conditions might progress over time. For instance, incorporating genetic information could help identify patients at higher risk for conditions like AMD or DR long before clinical symptoms appear, allowing for earlier and more targeted interventions [42,52]. Additionally, leveraging patient history data, including previous treatments, outcomes, and other health conditions, can further refine AI models. This approach enables the creation of personalized treatment plans that account for a patient's unique medical background, improving the accuracy and effectiveness of care. For example, in managing glaucoma, an AI system that considers a patient's comprehensive medical history could better predict disease progression and suggest personalized treatment adjustments, enhancing overall patient outcomes [64].

Developing advanced AI models will require collaboration across multiple disciplines [125], including ophthalmology, genetics, bioinformatics, and computer science. Researchers will need to address several technical challenges, such as ensuring data interoperability, managing large and complex datasets, and developing algorithms that can seamlessly integrate and analyze multimodal data. Moreover, ethical considerations, such as patient consent for the use of genetic data and the potential for genetic discrimination, must be carefully managed to ensure patient trust and regulatory compliance. By focusing on these future directions, the field of ophthalmology can harness AI's full potential, leading to more precise diagnoses, personalized treatments, and, ultimately, better patient outcomes. As AI models become increasingly sophisticated and capable of integrating diverse data sources, they will play a crucial role in advancing ophthalmic care and research.

7.2. Global Health Initiatives

AI-driven teleophthalmology services hold immense potential for addressing global eye health challenges, particularly in low-resource settings. These services leverage AI technologies to screen for and diagnose eye diseases remotely, thereby overcoming geographical and infrastructural barriers that often limit access to quality eye care. By expanding the reach of teleophthalmology, AI can play a pivotal role in improving eye health outcomes on a global scale. In low-resource settings, the scarcity of trained ophthalmologists and advanced medical facilities significantly hampers the delivery of eye care. AI-driven teleophthalmology can mitigate these issues by providing accurate, real-time screening and diagnostic capabilities via mobile devices and internet platforms. For instance, AI algorithms can analyze retinal images taken with portable fundus cameras and identify signs of DR, glaucoma, or other eye conditions with high accuracy. Patients in remote areas can then receive timely referrals and follow-up care, which is critical for preventing vision loss and managing chronic eye diseases.

To effectively deploy AI solutions in low-resource settings, collaborative efforts between governments, NGOs, and technology companies are essential. Governments can play a crucial role by creating supportive policies and frameworks that facilitate the integration of AI in healthcare systems [126]. This includes investing in digital infrastructure, ensuring data privacy and security, and providing funding for AI-based health initiatives. NGOs, which often work on the ground in underserved communities, can help implement and scale AI-driven teleophthalmology programs. Their deep understanding of local health challenges and trust within the communities they serve make them valuable partners in these initiatives. NGOs can assist in training local healthcare workers to use AI tools, raising awareness about the importance of eye health, and facilitating the logistics of teleophthalmology services. Technology companies bring the necessary expertise in AI development and deployment. By collaborating with healthcare providers and NGOs, they can tailor AI solutions to meet the specific needs of different populations. For example, companies can develop user-friendly AI applications that are accessible to healthcare workers with varying levels of technical expertise. Moreover, these companies can provide ongoing technical support and updates to ensure that AI systems remain effective and up to date with the latest medical standards and practices.

The expansion of AI-driven teleophthalmology services can significantly improve access to quality eye care worldwide. In regions where traditional healthcare infrastructure is lacking, these services offer a practical and scalable solution to bridge the gap. For example, in rural and underserved urban areas, AI-powered mobile clinics can provide essential eye care services, reducing the burden of travel for patients and making it easier for them to receive timely and effective treatment. Furthermore, by enabling early detection and intervention, AI-driven teleophthalmology can help reduce the prevalence of preventable blindness and vision impairment. Early diagnosis of conditions such as DR or glaucoma can lead to better management and treatment outcomes, ultimately preserving vision and enhancing the quality of life for patients. This proactive approach not only benefits individual patients but also alleviates the broader economic and social burden associated with vision loss.

8. Limitations of the Review

While this narrative review provides a comprehensive overview of current AI applications in ophthalmology, it has several limitations. First, due to language constraints, only articles published in English were included, which may have led to the exclusion of relevant studies from key regions such as Europe, China, and India where AI research is rapidly emerging. Although modern translation tools (e.g., Google Translate) are available, their use was not employed in this review, potentially limiting the scope of the evidence considered. Second, as a narrative review, the quality of the included articles was not formally evaluated using systematic criteria such as a PICO strategy, which is essential for assessing the strength of evidence in systematic reviews. Consequently, the conclusions drawn from this review may lack the rigorous quality appraisal that is necessary for evidence-based practice. Future work should consider incorporating non-English literature and employing systematic quality assessment methods to further enhance the robustness and generalizability of the findings.

9. Conclusions

AI is poised to revolutionize ophthalmology by enhancing diagnostic accuracy, personalizing treatment, and improving service delivery. The application of AI in ophthalmology encompasses a wide range of innovations, from advanced diagnostic tools that can detect conditions like DR, age-related macular degeneration, and glaucoma with remarkable precision to personalized treatment plans that optimize therapeutic outcomes and reduce costs. Additionally, AI-driven surgical tools and teleophthalmology services are making high-quality eye care more accessible, particularly in underserved and remote areas. Despite these promising advancements, several challenges need to be addressed to fully integrate AI into ophthalmic practice. Data privacy and security remain paramount concerns, necessitating robust encryption methods, stringent access controls, and comprehensive data governance frameworks. Addressing algorithmic biases is also crucial to ensure that

AI systems provide equitable care across diverse patient populations. Furthermore, interoperability issues and the need for user acceptance highlight the importance of training healthcare professionals and designing user-friendly AI solutions.

The potential benefits of AI in ophthalmology are immense. By continuing to invest in research and development, fostering ethical practices, and encouraging collaborative efforts between technologists, clinicians, and policymakers, the ophthalmic community can overcome these challenges. Such collaborative efforts are essential to develop and deploy AI systems that are both effective and ethically sound. As AI technology evolves, it holds the promise of transforming ophthalmic care, leading to better patient outcomes, more efficient clinical workflows, and broader access to high-quality eye care services globally. By harnessing the power of AI, we can make significant strides toward improving vision health and preventing blindness on a global scale.

Author Contributions: Conceptualization, D.B.O. and K.W.; methodology, M.D.D.E.M.; software, A.O.; validation, N.A. and J.T.; formal analysis, M.D.D.E.M.; investigation, N.A.; resources, K.W.; data curation, D.B.O. and S.B.; writing—original draft preparation, D.B.O. and K.W.; writing—review and editing, D.B.O., K.W., M.D.D.E.M., A.O., N.A., J.T. and S.B.; visualization, D.B.O.; supervision, S.B.; project administration, J.T.; funding acquisition, S.B. All authors have read and agreed to the published version of the manuscript.

Funding: This research received no external funding.

Acknowledgments: The work was supported by the Department of Research and Innovation, Medway NHS Foundation Trust, Gillingham, Kent, UK.

Conflicts of Interest: The authors declare no conflicts of interest.

References

1. Matcha, A. Innovations in Healthcare: Transforming Patient Care through Technology, Personalized Medicine, and Global Health Crises. *IJSR* **2023**, *12*, 1668–1672. [CrossRef]
2. Redd, T.K.; Al-Khaled, T.; Paul Chan, R.V.; Campbell, J.P. Technology and Innovation in Global Ophthalmology: The Past, the Potential, and a Path Forward. *Int. Ophthalmol. Clin.* **2023**, *63*, 25–32. [CrossRef] [PubMed]
3. Bhatia, R. Emerging Health Technologies and How They Can Transform Healthcare Delivery. *J. Health Manag.* **2021**, *23*, 63–73. [CrossRef]
4. Pinto-Coelho, L. How Artificial Intelligence Is Shaping Medical Imaging Technology: A Survey of Innovations and Applications. *Bioengineering* **2023**, *10*, 1435. [CrossRef]
5. Oren, O.; Gersh, B.J.; Bhatt, D.L. Artificial intelligence in medical imaging: Switching from radiographic pathological data to clinically meaningful endpoints. *Lancet Digit. Health* **2020**, *2*, e486–e488. [CrossRef] [PubMed]
6. Shehab, M.; Abualigah, L.; Shambour, Q.; Abu-Hashem, M.A.; Shambour, M.K.Y.; Alsalibi, A.I.; Gandomi, A.H. Machine learning in medical applications: A review of state-of-the-art methods. *Comput. Biol. Med.* **2022**, *145*, 105458. [CrossRef] [PubMed]
7. Alzubaidi, L.; Zhang, J.; Humaidi, A.J.; Al-Dujaili, A.; Duan, Y.; Al-Shamma, O.; Santamaría, J.; Fadhel, M.A.; Al-Amidie, M.; Farhan, L. Review of deep learning: Concepts, CNN architectures, challenges, applications, future directions. *J. Big Data* **2021**, *8*, 53. [CrossRef] [PubMed]
8. Tan, T.F.; Thirunavukarasu, A.J.; Jin, L.; Lim, J.; Poh, S.; Teo, Z.L.; Ang, M.; Chan, R.V.P.; Ong, J.; Turner, A.; et al. Artificial intelligence and digital health in global eye health: Opportunities and challenges. *Lancet Glob. Health* **2023**, *11*, e1432–e1443. [CrossRef] [PubMed]
9. Abràmoff, M.D.; Lavin, P.T.; Birch, M.; Shah, N.; Folk, J.C. Pivotal trial of an autonomous AI-based diagnostic system for detection of diabetic retinopathy in primary care offices. *NPJ Digit. Med.* **2018**, *1*, 39. [CrossRef]
10. Gulshan, V.; Peng, L.; Coram, M.; Stumpe, M.C.; Wu, D.; Narayanaswamy, A.; Venugopalan, S.; Widner, K.; Madams, T.; Cuadros, J.; et al. Development and Validation of a Deep Learning Algorithm for Detection of Diabetic Retinopathy in Retinal Fundus Photographs. *JAMA* **2016**, *316*, 2402–2410. [CrossRef] [PubMed]
11. Schmidt-Erfurth, U.; Sadeghipour, A.; Gerendas, B.S.; Waldstein, S.M.; Bogunović, H. Artificial intelligence in retina. *Prog. Retin. Eye Res.* **2018**, *67*, 1–29. [CrossRef]

12. De Fauw, J.; Ledsam, J.R.; Romera-Paredes, B.; Nikolov, S.; Tomasev, N.; Blackwell, S.; Askham, H.; Glorot, X.; O'Donoghue, B.; Visentin, D.; et al. Clinically applicable deep learning for diagnosis and referral in retinal disease. *Nat. Med.* **2018**, *24*, 1342–1350. [CrossRef] [PubMed]
13. Kropp, M.; Golubnitschaja, O.; Mazurakova, A.; Koklesova, L.; Sargheini, N.; Vo, T.K.S.; de Clerck, E.; Polivka, J., Jr.; Potuznik, P.; Polivka, J.; et al. Diabetic retinopathy as the leading cause of blindness and early predictor of cascading complications-risks and mitigation. *EPMA J.* **2023**, *14*, 21–42. [CrossRef] [PubMed]
14. Burlina, P.M.; Joshi, N.; Pekala, M.; Pacheco, K.D.; Freund, D.E.; Bressler, N.M. Automated Grading of Age-Related Macular Degeneration From Color Fundus Images Using Deep Convolutional Neural Networks. *JAMA Ophthalmol.* **2017**, *135*, 1170–1176. [CrossRef] [PubMed]
15. Jonas, J.B.; Aung, T.; Bourne, R.R.; Bron, A.M.; Ritch, R.; Panda-Jonas, S. Glaucoma. *Lancet* **2017**, *390*, 2183–2193. [CrossRef] [PubMed]
16. Weinreb, R.N.; Aung, T.; Medeiros, F.A. The pathophysiology and treatment of glaucoma: A review. *JAMA* **2014**, *311*, 1901–1911. [CrossRef]
17. Zhu, Y.; Salowe, R.; Chow, C.; Li, S.; Bastani, O.; O'Brien, J.M. Advancing Glaucoma Care: Integrating Artificial Intelligence in Diagnosis, Management, and Progression Detection. *Bioengineering* **2024**, *11*, 122. [CrossRef]
18. Christopher, M.; Belghith, A.; Bowd, C.; Proudfoot, J.A.; Goldbaum, M.H.; Weinreb, R.N.; Girkin, C.A.; Liebmann, J.M.; Zangwill, L.M. Performance of Deep Learning Architectures and Transfer Learning for Detecting Glaucomatous Optic Neuropathy in Fundus Photographs. *Sci. Rep.* **2018**, *8*, 16685. [CrossRef]
19. Topol, E.J. High-performance medicine: The convergence of human and artificial intelligence. *Nat. Med.* **2019**, *25*, 44–56. [CrossRef]
20. Yu, K.H.; Beam, A.L.; Kohane, I.S. Artificial intelligence in healthcare. *Nat. Biomed. Eng.* **2018**, *2*, 719–731. [CrossRef] [PubMed]
21. Yelne, S.; Chaudhary, M.; Dod, K.; Sayyad, A.; Sharma, R. Harnessing the Power of AI: A Comprehensive Review of Its Impact and Challenges in Nursing Science and Healthcare. *Cureus* **2023**, *15*, e49252. [CrossRef] [PubMed]
22. Alowais, S.A.; Alghamdi, S.S.; Alsuhebany, N.; Alqahtani, T.; Alshaya, A.I.; Almohareb, S.N.; Aldairem, A.; Alrashed, M.; Bin Saleh, K.; Badreldin, H.A.; et al. Revolutionizing healthcare: The role of artificial intelligence in clinical practice. *BMC Med. Educ.* **2023**, *23*, 689. [CrossRef] [PubMed]
23. Wolf, R.M.; Channa, R.; Liu, T.Y.A.; Zehra, A.; Bromberger, L.; Patel, D.; Ananthakrishnan, A.; Brown, E.A.; Prichett, L.; Lehmann, H.P.; et al. Autonomous artificial intelligence increases screening and follow-up for diabetic retinopathy in youth: The ACCESS randomized control trial. *Nat. Commun.* **2024**, *15*, 421. [CrossRef] [PubMed]
24. Campbell, J.P.; Mathenge, C.; Cherwek, H.; Balaskas, K.; Pasquale, L.R.; Keane, P.A.; Chiang, M.F. Artificial Intelligence to Reduce Ocular Health Disparities: Moving From Concept to Implementation. *Transl. Vis. Sci. Technol.* **2021**, *10*, 19. [CrossRef] [PubMed]
25. Joseph, S.; Selvaraj, J.; Mani, I.; Kumaragurupari, T.; Shang, X.; Mudgil, P.; Ravilla, T.; He, M. Diagnostic Accuracy of Artificial Intelligence-Based Automated Diabetic Retinopathy Screening in Real-World Settings: A Systematic Review and Meta-Analysis. *Am. J. Ophthalmol.* **2024**, *263*, 214–230. [CrossRef] [PubMed]
26. Chokshi, T.; Cruz, M.J.; Ross, J.; You, G. Advances in teleophthalmology and artificial intelligence for diabetic retinopathy screening: A narrative review. *Ann. Eye Sci.* **2024**, *9*, 9. [CrossRef]
27. Pieczynski, J.; Kuklo, P.; Grzybowski, A. The Role of Telemedicine, In-Home Testing and Artificial Intelligence to Alleviate an Increasingly Burdened Healthcare System: Diabetic Retinopathy. *Ophthalmol. Ther.* **2021**, *10*, 445–464. [CrossRef] [PubMed]
28. Mursch-Edlmayr, A.S.; Ng, W.S.; Diniz-Filho, A.; Sousa, D.C.; Arnold, L.; Schlenker, M.B.; Duenas-Angeles, K.; Keane, P.A.; Crowston, J.G.; Jayaram, H. Artificial Intelligence Algorithms to Diagnose Glaucoma and Detect Glaucoma Progression: Translation to Clinical Practice. *Transl. Vis. Sci. Technol.* **2020**, *9*, 55. [CrossRef]
29. Shimizu, E.; Tanji, M.; Nakayama, S.; Ishikawa, T.; Agata, N.; Yokoiwa, R.; Nishimura, H.; Khemlani, R.J.; Sato, S.; Hanyuda, A.; et al. AI-based diagnosis of nuclear cataract from slit-lamp videos. *Sci. Rep.* **2023**, *13*, 22046. [CrossRef]
30. Son, K.Y.; Ko, J.; Kim, E.; Lee, S.Y.; Kim, M.J.; Han, J.; Shin, E.; Chung, T.Y.; Lim, D.H. Deep Learning-Based Cataract Detection and Grading from Slit-Lamp and Retro-Illumination Photographs: Model Development and Validation Study. *Ophthalmol. Sci.* **2022**, *2*, 100147. [CrossRef]
31. Ji, Y.K.; Hua, R.R.; Liu, S.; Xie, C.J.; Zhang, S.C.; Yang, W.H. Intelligent diagnosis of retinal vein occlusion based on color fundus photographs. *Int. J. Ophthalmol.* **2024**, *17*, 1–6. [CrossRef]
32. Huang, S.; Jin, K.; Gao, Z.; Yang, B.; Shi, X.; Zhou, J.; Grzybowski, A.; Gawecki, M.; Ye, J. Automated interpretation of retinal vein occlusion based on fundus fluorescein angiography images using deep learning: A retrospective, multi-center study. *Heliyon* **2024**, *10*, e33108. [CrossRef]
33. Parmar, U.P.S.; Surico, P.L.; Singh, R.B.; Romano, F.; Salati, C.; Spadea, L.; Musa, M.; Gagliano, C.; Mori, T.; Zeppieri, M. Artificial Intelligence (AI) for Early Diagnosis of Retinal Diseases. *Medicina* **2024**, *60*, 527. [CrossRef] [PubMed]

34. Chen, T.C.; Lim, W.S.; Wang, V.Y.; Ko, M.L.; Chiu, S.I.; Huang, Y.S.; Lai, F.; Yang, C.M.; Hu, F.R.; Jang, J.R.; et al. Artificial Intelligence-Assisted Early Detection of Retinitis Pigmentosa—The Most Common Inherited Retinal Degeneration. *J. Digit. Imaging* **2021**, *34*, 948–958. [CrossRef] [PubMed]
35. Niazi, S.; Jiménez-García, M.; Findl, O.; Gatzioufas, Z.; Doroodgar, F.; Shahriari, M.H.; Javadi, M.A. Keratoconus Diagnosis: From Fundamentals to Artificial Intelligence: A Systematic Narrative Review. *Diagnostics* **2023**, *13*, 2715. [CrossRef] [PubMed]
36. Ji, Y.; Liu, S.; Hong, X.; Lu, Y.; Wu, X.; Li, K.; Li, K.; Liu, Y. Advances in artificial intelligence applications for ocular surface diseases diagnosis. *Front. Cell Dev. Biol.* **2022**, *10*, 1107689. [CrossRef] [PubMed]
37. Nakayama, L.F.; Ribeiro, L.Z.; Dychiao, R.G.; Zamora, Y.F.; Regatieri, C.V.S.; Celi, L.A.; Silva, P.; Sobrin, L.; Belfort, R., Jr. Artificial intelligence in uveitis: A comprehensive review. *Surv. Ophthalmol.* **2023**, *68*, 669–677. [CrossRef] [PubMed]
38. Jacquot, R.; Sève, P.; Jackson, T.L.; Wang, T.; Duclos, A.; Stanescu-Segall, D. Diagnosis, Classification, and Assessment of the Underlying Etiology of Uveitis by Artificial Intelligence: A Systematic Review. *J. Clin. Med.* **2023**, *12*, 3746. [CrossRef]
39. Mennella, C.; Maniscalco, U.; De Pietro, G.; Esposito, M. Ethical and regulatory challenges of AI technologies in healthcare: A narrative review. *Heliyon* **2024**, *10*, e26297. [CrossRef] [PubMed]
40. Hou, X.; Wang, L.; Zhu, D.; Guo, L.; Weng, J.; Zhang, M.; Zhou, Z.; Zou, D.; Ji, Q.; Guo, X.; et al. Prevalence of diabetic retinopathy and vision-threatening diabetic retinopathy in adults with diabetes in China. *Nat. Commun.* **2023**, *14*, 4296. [CrossRef] [PubMed]
41. Teo, Z.L.; Tham, Y.C.; Yu, M.; Chee, M.L.; Rim, T.H.; Cheung, N.; Bikbov, M.M.; Wang, Y.X.; Tang, Y.; Lu, Y.; et al. Global Prevalence of Diabetic Retinopathy and Projection of Burden through 2045: Systematic Review and Meta-analysis. *Ophthalmology* **2021**, *128*, 1580–1591. [CrossRef] [PubMed]
42. Kong, M.; Song, S.J. Artificial Intelligence Applications in Diabetic Retinopathy: What We Have Now and What to Expect in the Future. *Endocrinol. Metab.* **2024**, *39*, 416–424. [CrossRef]
43. Gargeya, R.; Leng, T. Automated Identification of Diabetic Retinopathy Using Deep Learning. *Ophthalmology* **2017**, *124*, 962–969. [CrossRef] [PubMed]
44. Pandey, P.U.; Ballios, B.G.; Christakis, P.G.; Kaplan, A.J.; Mathew, D.J.; Ong Tone, S.; Wan, M.J.; Micieli, J.A.; Wong, J.C.Y. Ensemble of deep convolutional neural networks is more accurate and reliable than board-certified ophthalmologists at detecting multiple diseases in retinal fundus photographs. *Br. J. Ophthalmol.* **2024**, *108*, 417–423. [CrossRef] [PubMed]
45. Ting, D.S.W.; Cheung, C.Y.; Lim, G.; Tan, G.S.W.; Quang, N.D.; Gan, A.; Hamzah, H.; Garcia-Franco, R.; San Yeo, I.Y.; Lee, S.Y.; et al. Development and Validation of a Deep Learning System for Diabetic Retinopathy and Related Eye Diseases Using Retinal Images From Multiethnic Populations With Diabetes. *JAMA* **2017**, *318*, 2211–2223. [CrossRef]
46. Rajalakshmi, R.; Subashini, R.; Anjana, R.M.; Mohan, V. Automated diabetic retinopathy detection in smartphone-based fundus photography using artificial intelligence. *Eye* **2018**, *32*, 1138–1144. [CrossRef]
47. Gulshan, V.; Rajan, R.P.; Widner, K.; Wu, D.; Wubbels, P.; Rhodes, T.; Whitehouse, K.; Coram, M.; Corrado, G.; Ramasamy, K.; et al. Performance of a Deep-Learning Algorithm vs Manual Grading for Detecting Diabetic Retinopathy in India. *JAMA Ophthalmol.* **2019**, *137*, 987–993. [CrossRef] [PubMed]
48. Fleckenstein, M.; Schmitz-Valckenberg, S.; Chakravarthy, U. Age-Related Macular Degeneration: A Review. *JAMA* **2024**, *331*, 147–157. [CrossRef]
49. Elsharkawy, M.; Elrazzaz, M.; Ghazal, M.; Alhalabi, M.; Soliman, A.; Mahmoud, A.; El-Daydamony, E.; Atwan, A.; Thanos, A.; Sandhu, H.S.; et al. Role of Optical Coherence Tomography Imaging in Predicting Progression of Age-Related Macular Disease: A Survey. *Diagnostics* **2021**, *11*, 2313. [CrossRef] [PubMed]
50. Arabi, P.M.; Krishna, N.; Ashwini, V.; Prathibha, H.M. Identification of Age-Related Macular Degeneration Using OCT Images. *IOP Conf. Ser. Mater. Sci. Eng.* **2018**, *310*, 012096. [CrossRef]
51. Kermany, D.S.; Goldbaum, M.; Cai, W.; Valentim, C.C.S.; Liang, H.; Baxter, S.L.; McKeown, A.; Yang, G.; Wu, X.; Yan, F.; et al. Identifying Medical Diagnoses and Treatable Diseases by Image-Based Deep Learning. *Cell* **2018**, *172*, 1122–1131.e9. [CrossRef] [PubMed]
52. Muntean, G.A.; Marginean, A.; Groza, A.; Damian, I.; Roman, S.A.; Hapca, M.C.; Muntean, M.V.; Nicoară, S.D. The Predictive Capabilities of Artificial Intelligence-Based OCT Analysis for Age-Related Macular Degeneration Progression-A Systematic Review. *Diagnostics* **2023**, *13*, 2464. [CrossRef] [PubMed]
53. Thakoor, K.A.; Yao, J.; Bordbar, D.; Moussa, O.; Lin, W.; Sajda, P.; Chen, R.W.S. A multimodal deep learning system to distinguish late stages of AMD and to compare expert vs. AI ocular biomarkers. *Sci. Rep.* **2022**, *12*, 2585. [CrossRef]
54. Mares, V.; Nehemy, M.B.; Bogunovic, H.; Frank, S.; Reiter, G.S.; Schmidt-Erfurth, U. AI-based support for optical coherence tomography in age-related macular degeneration. *Int. J. Retin. Vitr.* **2024**, *10*, 31. [CrossRef]
55. Saleh, G.A.; Batouty, N.M.; Haggag, S.; Elnakib, A.; Khalifa, F.; Taher, F.; Mohamed, M.A.; Farag, R.; Sandhu, H.; Sewelam, A.; et al. The Role of Medical Image Modalities and AI in the Early Detection, Diagnosis and Grading of Retinal Diseases: A Survey. *Bioengineering* **2022**, *9*, 366. [CrossRef] [PubMed]

56. Yim, J.; Chopra, R.; De Fauw, J.; Ledsam, J. Using AI to Predict Retinal Disease Progression. Google DeepMind. Published 18 May 2020. Available online: https://deepmind.google/discover/blog/using-ai-to-predict-retinal-disease-progression/ (accessed on 25 July 2024).
57. Lee, C.S.; Tyring, A.J.; Deruyter, N.P.; Wu, Y.; Rokem, A.; Lee, A.Y. Deep-learning based, automated segmentation of macular edema in optical coherence tomography. *Biomed. Opt. Express* **2017**, *8*, 3440–3448. [CrossRef] [PubMed]
58. Liu, X.; Zhao, C.; Wang, L.; Wang, G.; Lv, B.; Lv, C.; Xie, G.; Wang, F. Evaluation of an OCT-AI-Based Telemedicine Platform for Retinal Disease Screening and Referral in a Primary Care Setting. *Transl. Vis. Sci. Technol.* **2022**, *11*, 4. [CrossRef] [PubMed]
59. Mantena, S.; Celi, L.A.; Keshavjee, S.; Beratarrechea, A. Improving community health-care screenings with smartphone-based AI technologies. *Lancet Digit. Health* **2021**, *3*, e280–e282. [CrossRef]
60. Allison, K.; Patel, D.; Alabi, O. Epidemiology of Glaucoma: The Past, Present, and Predictions for the Future. *Cureus* **2020**, *12*, e11686. [CrossRef] [PubMed]
61. Tham, Y.C.; Li, X.; Wong, T.Y.; Quigley, H.A.; Aung, T.; Cheng, C.Y. Global prevalence of glaucoma and projections of glaucoma burden through 2040: A systematic review and meta-analysis. *Ophthalmology* **2014**, *121*, 2081–2090. [CrossRef]
62. Bragança, C.P.; Torres, J.M.; Macedo, L.O.; Soares, C.P.A. Advancements in Glaucoma Diagnosis: The Role of AI in Medical Imaging. *Diagnostics* **2024**, *14*, 530. [CrossRef] [PubMed]
63. Yousefi, S. Clinical Applications of Artificial Intelligence in Glaucoma. *J. Ophthalmic. Vis. Res.* **2023**, *18*, 97–112. [CrossRef] [PubMed]
64. Zhang, L.; Tang, L.; Xia, M.; Cao, G. The application of artificial intelligence in glaucoma diagnosis and prediction. *Front. Cell Dev. Biol.* **2023**, *11*, 1173094. [CrossRef] [PubMed]
65. Turbert, D. Visual Field Test. American Academy of Ophthalmology. Published 27 January 2022. Available online: https://www.aao.org/eye-health/tips-prevention/visual-field-testing (accessed on 26 July 2024).
66. Broadway, D.C. Visual field testing for glaucoma—A practical guide. *Community Eye Health* **2012**, *25*, 66–70. [PubMed]
67. AlShawabkeh, M.; AlRyalat, S.A.; Al Bdour, M.; Alni'mat, A.; Al-Akhras, M. The utilization of artificial intelligence in glaucoma: Diagnosis versus screening. *Front. Ophthalmol.* **2024**, *4*, 1368081. [CrossRef] [PubMed]
68. Hussain, S.; Chua, J.; Wong, D.; Lo, J.; Kadziauskiene, A.; Asoklis, R.; Barbastathis, G.; Schmetterer, L.; Yong, L. Predicting glaucoma progression using deep learning framework guided by generative algorithm. *Sci. Rep.* **2023**, *13*, 19960. [CrossRef]
69. Medeiros, F.A.; Jammal, A.A.; Thompson, A.C. From Machine to Machine: An OCT-Trained Deep Learning Algorithm for Objective Quantification of Glaucomatous Damage in Fundus Photographs. *Ophthalmology* **2019**, *126*, 513–521. [CrossRef] [PubMed]
70. Bhartiya, S. Glaucoma Screening: Is AI the Answer? *J. Curr. Glaucoma Pract.* **2022**, *16*, 71–73. [CrossRef]
71. Krishnan, G.; Singh, S.; Pathania, M.; Gosavi, S.; Abhishek, S.; Parchani, A.; Dhar, M. Artificial intelligence in clinical medicine: Catalyzing a sustainable global healthcare paradigm. *Front. Artif. Intell.* **2023**, *6*, 1227091. [CrossRef] [PubMed]
72. Meng, Z.; Chen, Y.; Li, H.; Zhang, Y.; Yao, X.; Meng, Y.; Shi, W.; Liang, Y.; Hu, Y.; Liu, D.; et al. Machine learning and optical coherence tomography-derived radiomics analysis to predict persistent diabetic macular edema in patients undergoing anti-VEGF intravitreal therapy. *J. Transl. Med.* **2024**, *22*, 358. [CrossRef]
73. Khalifa, M.; Albadawy, M. Artificial Intelligence for Clinical Prediction: Exploring Key Domains and Essential Functions. *Comput. Methods Programs Biomed. Update* **2024**, *5*, 100148. [CrossRef]
74. Khansari, N. AI machine learning improves personalized cancer therapies. *AMJ* **2024**, *17*, 1166–1173. [CrossRef]
75. Nuliqiman, M.; Xu, M.; Sun, Y.; Cao, J.; Chen, P.; Gao, Q.; Xu, P.; Ye, J. Artificial Intelligence in Ophthalmic Surgery: Current Applications and Expectations. *Clin. Ophthalmol.* **2023**, *17*, 3499–3511. [CrossRef] [PubMed]
76. Alafaleq, M. Robotics and cybersurgery in ophthalmology: A current perspective. *J. Robot. Surg.* **2023**, *17*, 1159–1170. [CrossRef] [PubMed]
77. Lindegger, D.J.; Wawrzynski, J.; Saleh, G.M. Evolution and Applications of Artificial Intelligence to Cataract Surgery. *Ophthalmol. Sci.* **2022**, *2*, 100164. [CrossRef] [PubMed]
78. Wang, T.; Xia, J.; Jin, L.; Zeng, D.; Yan, P.; Lin, S.; Huang, K.; Lin, H. Comparison of robot-assisted vitreoretinal surgery and manual surgery in different preclinical settings: A randomized trial. *Ann. Transl. Med.* **2022**, *10*, 1163. [CrossRef] [PubMed]
79. Pandey, S.K.; Sharma, V. Robotics and ophthalmology: Are we there yet? *Indian J. Ophthalmol.* **2019**, *67*, 988–994. [CrossRef] [PubMed]
80. de Smet, M.D.; Naus, G.J.L.; Faridpooya, K.; Mura, M. Robotic-assisted surgery in ophthalmology. *Curr. Opin. Ophthalmol.* **2018**, *29*, 248–253. [CrossRef]
81. Reddy, K.; Gharde, P.; Tayade, H.; Patil, M.; Reddy, L.S.; Surya, D. Advancements in Robotic Surgery: A Comprehensive Overview of Current Utilizations and Upcoming Frontiers. *Cureus* **2023**, *15*, e50415. [CrossRef]
82. Roberts, H.W.; Day, A.C.; O'Brart, D.P. Femtosecond laser-assisted cataract surgery: A review. *Eur. J. Ophthalmol.* **2020**, *30*, 417–429. [CrossRef]

83. Müller, S.; Jain, M.; Sachdeva, B.; Shah, P.N.; Holz, F.G.; Finger, R.P.; Murali, K.; Wintergerst, M.W.M.; Schultz, T. Artificial Intelligence in Cataract Surgery: A Systematic Review. *Transl. Vis. Sci. Technol.* **2024**, *13*, 20. [CrossRef]
84. Li, Z.; Wang, L.; Wu, X.; Jiang, J.; Qiang, W.; Xie, H.; Zhou, H.; Wu, S.; Shao, Y.; Chen, W. Artificial intelligence in ophthalmology: The path to the real-world clinic. *Cell Rep. Med.* **2023**, *4*, 101095. [CrossRef] [PubMed]
85. Kecik, M.; Schweitzer, C. Femtosecond laser-assisted cataract surgery: Update and perspectives. *Front. Med.* **2023**, *10*, 1131314. [CrossRef] [PubMed]
86. Koetting, C. All eyes on the future: How AI is revolutionizing ocular surgery. *Optom. Times* **2024**, *16*, 24–25. Available online: https://www.optometrytimes.com/view/all-eyes-on-the-future-how-ai-is-revolutionizing-ocular-surgery (accessed on 25 February 2025).
87. Skevas, C.; de Olaguer, N.P.; Lleó, A.; Thiwa, D.; Schroeter, U.; Lopes, I.V.; Mautone, L.; Linke, S.J.; Spitzer, M.S.; Yap, D.; et al. Implementing and evaluating a fully functional AI-enabled model for chronic eye disease screening in a real clinical environment. *BMC Ophthalmol.* **2024**, *24*, 51. [CrossRef]
88. Swaminathan, U.; Daigavane, S. Unveiling the Potential: A Comprehensive Review of Artificial Intelligence Applications in Ophthalmology and Future Prospects. *Cureus* **2024**, *16*, e61826. [CrossRef]
89. Wang, Y.; Liu, C.; Hu, W.; Luo, L.; Shi, D.; Zhang, J.; Yin, Q.; Zhang, L.; Han, X.; He, M. Economic evaluation for medical artificial intelligence: Accuracy vs. cost-effectiveness in a diabetic retinopathy screening case. *NPJ Digit. Med.* **2024**, *7*, 43. [CrossRef] [PubMed]
90. Jin, K.; Li, Y.; Wu, H.; Tham, Y.C.; Koh, V.; Zhao, Y.; Kawasaki, R.; Grzybowski, A.; Ye, J. Integration of smartphone technology and artificial intelligence for advanced ophthalmic care: A systematic review. *Adv. Ophthalmol. Pract. Res.* **2024**, *4*, 120–127. [CrossRef] [PubMed]
91. Chia, M.A.; Turner, A.W. Benefits of Integrating Telemedicine and Artificial Intelligence Into Outreach Eye Care: Stepwise Approach and Future Directions. *Front. Med.* **2022**, *9*, 835804. [CrossRef] [PubMed]
92. Gupta, V.; Azad, S.V.; Vashist, P.; Senjam, S.S.; Kumar, A. Diabetic retinopathy screening in the public sector in India: What is needed? *Indian J. Ophthalmol.* **2022**, *70*, 759–767. [CrossRef]
93. Cuadros, J.; Bresnick, G. EyePACS: An adaptable telemedicine system for diabetic retinopathy screening. *J. Diabetes Sci. Technol.* **2009**, *3*, 509–516. [CrossRef] [PubMed]
94. Maleki Varnosfaderani, S.; Forouzanfar, M. The Role of AI in Hospitals and Clinics: Transforming Healthcare in the 21st Century. *Bioengineering* **2024**, *11*, 337. [CrossRef] [PubMed]
95. Marchiori, C.; Dykeman, D.; Girardi, I.; Ivankay, A.; Thandiackal, K.; Zusag, M.; Giovannini, A.; Karpati, D.; Saenz, H. Artificial Intelligence Decision Support for Medical Triage. *AMIA Annu. Symp. Proc.* **2021**, *2020*, 793–802.
96. Evans, N.G.; Wenner, D.M.; Cohen, I.G.; Purves, D.; Chiang, M.F.; Ting, D.S.W.; Lee, A.Y. Emerging Ethical Considerations for the Use of Artificial Intelligence in Ophthalmology. *Ophthalmol. Sci.* **2022**, *2*, 100141. [CrossRef] [PubMed]
97. Tom, E.; Keane, P.A.; Blazes, M.; Pasquale, L.R.; Chiang, M.F.; Lee, A.Y.; Lee, C.S. Protecting Data Privacy in the Age of AI-Enabled Ophthalmology. *Transl. Vis. Sci. Technol.* **2020**, *9*, 36. [CrossRef]
98. Zarour, M.; Alenezi, M.; Ansari, M.T.J.; Pandey, A.K.; Ahmad, M.; Agrawal, A.; Kumar, R.; Khan, R.A. Ensuring data integrity of healthcare information in the era of digital health. *Healthc. Technol. Lett.* **2021**, *8*, 66–77. [CrossRef]
99. Adler-Milstein, J.; Adelman, J.S.; Tai-Seale, M.; Patel, V.L.; Dymek, C. EHR audit logs: A new goldmine for health services research? *J. Biomed. Inform.* **2020**, *101*, 103343. [CrossRef] [PubMed]
100. World Bank. Data Protection and Privacy Laws. Available online: https://id4d.worldbank.org/guide/data-protection-and-privacy-laws (accessed on 27 July 2024).
101. Jones, M.C.; Stone, T.; Mason, S.M.; Eames, A.; Franklin, M. Navigating data governance associated with real-world data for public benefit: An overview in the UK and future considerations. *BMJ Open* **2023**, *13*, e069925. [CrossRef] [PubMed]
102. Singhal, A.; Neveditsin, N.; Tanveer, H.; Mago, V. Toward Fairness, Accountability, Transparency, and Ethics in AI for Social Media and Health Care: Scoping Review. *JMIR Med. Inform.* **2024**, *12*, e50048. [CrossRef]
103. Al-Badi, A.; Tarhini, A.; Khan, A.I. Exploring Big Data Governance Frameworks. *Procedia Comput. Sci.* **2018**, *141*, 271–277. [CrossRef]
104. Neftenov, N.; Stankovic, M.; Gupta, R.; UNESCO. Data-Invisible Groups and Data Minimization in the Deployment of AI Solutions: Policy Brief. 2023, pp. 1–16. Available online: https://unesdoc.unesco.org/ark:/48223/pf0000388089 (accessed on 27 July 2024).
105. Zuo, Z.; Watson, M.; Budgen, D.; Hall, R.; Kennelly, C.; Al Moubayed, N. Data Anonymization for Pervasive Health Care: Systematic Literature Mapping Study. *JMIR Med. Inform.* **2021**, *9*, e29871. [CrossRef]
106. Puri, V.; Sachdeva, S.; Kaur, P. Privacy preserving publication of relational and transaction data: Survey on the anonymization of patient data. *Comput. Sci. Rev.* **2019**, *32*, 45–61. [CrossRef]
107. Yadav, N.; Pandey, S.; Gupta, A.; Dudani, P.; Gupta, S.; Rangarajan, K. Data Privacy in Healthcare: In the Era of Artificial Intelligence. *Indian Dermatol. Online J.* **2023**, *14*, 788–792. [CrossRef]

108. Gerke, S.; Minssen, T.; Cohen, G. Ethical and legal challenges of artificial intelligence-driven healthcare. In *Artificial Intelligence in Healthcare*; Academic Press: Cambridge, MA, USA, 2020; pp. 295–336. [CrossRef]
109. Friedewald, M.; Schiering, I.; Martin, N.; Hallinan, D. Data Protection Impact Assessments in Practice. In *Computer Security. ESORICS 2021 International Workshops. ESORICS 2021*; Lecture Notes in Computer Science; Springer: Cham, Switzerland, 2022; Volume 13106. [CrossRef]
110. Castillo, A.F.; Sirbu, M.; Davis, A.L. Vendor of choice and the effectiveness of policies to promote health information exchange. *BMC Health Serv. Res.* **2018**, *18*, 405. [CrossRef]
111. Char, D.S.; Shah, N.H.; Magnus, D. Implementing Machine Learning in Health Care—Addressing Ethical Challenges. *N. Engl. J. Med.* **2018**, *378*, 981–983. [CrossRef]
112. Mehrabi, N.; Morstatter, F.; Saxena, N.; Lerman, K.; Galstyan, A. A Survey on Bias and Fairness in Machine Learning. *ACM Comput. Surv.* **2021**, *54*, 1–35. [CrossRef]
113. Chen, I.Y.; Pierson, E.; Rose, S.; Joshi, S.; Ferryman, K.; Ghassemi, M. Ethical Machine Learning in Healthcare. *Annu. Rev. Biomed. Data Sci.* **2021**, *4*, 123–144. [CrossRef] [PubMed]
114. Gichoya, J.W.; Banerjee, I.; Bhimireddy, A.R.; Burns, J.L.; Celi, L.A.; Chen, L.C.; Correa, R.; Dullerud, N.; Ghassemi, M.; Huang, S.C.; et al. AI recognition of patient race in medical imaging: A modelling study. *Lancet Digit. Health* **2022**, *4*, e406–e414. [CrossRef] [PubMed]
115. Rajkomar, A.; Hardt, M.; Howell, M.D.; Corrado, G.; Chin, M.H. Ensuring Fairness in Machine Learning to Advance Health Equity. *Ann. Intern. Med.* **2018**, *169*, 866–872. [CrossRef]
116. Vokinger, K.N.; Feuerriegel, S.; Kesselheim, A.S. Mitigating bias in machine learning for medicine. *Commun. Med.* **2021**, *1*, 25. [CrossRef]
117. Ghassemi, M.; Naumann, T.; Schulam, P.; Beam, A.L.; Chen, I.Y.; Ranganath, R. A Review of Challenges and Opportunities in Machine Learning for Health. *AMIA Jt. Summits Transl. Sci. Proc.* **2020**, *2020*, 191–200. [PubMed]
118. Karalis, V.D. The Integration of Artificial Intelligence into Clinical Practice. *Appl. Biosci.* **2024**, *3*, 14–44. [CrossRef]
119. Keane, P.A.; Topol, E.J. AI-facilitated health care requires education of clinicians. *Lancet* **2021**, *397*, 1254. [CrossRef]
120. Tseng, R.M.W.W.; Gunasekeran, D.V.; Tan, S.S.H.; Rim, T.H.; Lum, E.; Tan, G.S.W.; Wong, T.Y.; Tham, Y.C. Considerations for Artificial Intelligence Real-World Implementation in Ophthalmology: Providers' and Patients' Perspectives. *Asia Pac. J. Ophthalmol.* **2021**, *10*, 299–306. [CrossRef] [PubMed]
121. Kinney, M.; Anastasiadou, M.; Naranjo-Zolotov, M.; Santos, V. Expectation management in AI: A framework for understanding stakeholder trust and acceptance of artificial intelligence systems. *Heliyon* **2024**, *10*, e28562. [CrossRef]
122. Kaye, J.; Shah, N.; Kogetsu, A.; Coy, S.; Katirai, A.; Kuroda, M.; Li, Y.; Kato, K.; Yamamoto, B.A. Moving beyond Technical Issues to Stakeholder Involvement: Key Areas for Consideration in the Development of Human-Centred and Trusted AI in Healthcare. *Asian Bioeth. Rev.* **2024**, *16*, 501–511. [CrossRef]
123. Dave, M.; Patel, N. Artificial intelligence in healthcare and education. *Br. Dent. J.* **2023**, *234*, 761–764. [CrossRef] [PubMed]
124. Olawade, D.B.; Teke, J.; Fapohunda, O.; Weerasinghe, K.; Usman, S.O.; Ige, A.O.; Clement David-Olawade, A. Leveraging artificial intelligence in vaccine development: A narrative review. *J. Microbiol. Methods* **2024**, *224*, 106998. [CrossRef] [PubMed]
125. Olawade, D.B.; Wada, O.J.; David-Olawade, A.C.; Kunonga, E.; Abaire, O.; Ling, J. Using artificial intelligence to improve public health: A narrative review. *Front. Public Health* **2023**, *11*, 1196397. [CrossRef] [PubMed]
126. Olawade, D.B.; David-Olawade, A.C.; Wada, O.Z.; Asaolu, A.J.; Adereni, T.; Ling, J. Artificial intelligence in healthcare delivery: Prospects and pitfalls. *J. Med. Surg. Public Health* **2024**, *3*, 100108. [CrossRef]

medicina

MDPI

Article

Non-Invasive Monitoring of Intracranial Pressure Pulse Waves from Closed Eyelids in Patients with Normal-Tension Glaucoma

Laimonas Bartusis [1,*], Solventa Krakauskaite [1], Ugne Kevalaite [2], Austeja Judickaite [2], Arminas Zizas [2], Akvile Stoskuviene [2,3], Edvinas Chaleckas [1], Mantas Deimantavicius [1], Yasin Hamarat [1], Fabien Scalzo [4], Kristina Berskiene [5], Ingrida Januleviciene [2] and Arminas Ragauskas [1]

1 Health Telematics Science Institute, Kaunas University of Technology, LT-51423 Kaunas, Lithuania; solventa@mail.com (S.K.); edvinas.chaleckas@ktu.lt (E.C.); m.deimantavicius@gmail.com (M.D.); yasin.hamarat@ktu.lt (Y.H.); arminas.ragauskas@ktu.lt (A.R.)
2 Eye Clinic, Lithuanian University of Health Sciences, LT-50161 Kaunas, Lithuania; ugne.kevalaite@lsmu.lt (U.K.); austeja.judickaite@lsmu.lt (A.J.); arminas.zizas@lsmu.lt (A.Z.); akvile.stoskuviene@lsmu.lt (A.S.); ingrida.januleviciene@kaunoklinikos.lt (I.J.)
3 Department of Neurology, Medical Academy, Lithuanian University of Health Sciences, LT-44037 Kaunas, Lithuania
4 Department of Neurology and Computer Science, University of California, Los Angeles (UCLA), Los Angeles, CA 90095, USA; fab@cs.ucla.edu
5 Department of Sports Medicine, Lithuanian University of Health Sciences, LT-50161, Kaunas, Lithuania; kristina.berskiene@lsmu.lt
* Correspondence: laimonas.bartusis@ktu.lt

Abstract: *Background and Objectives*: Normal-tension glaucoma (NTG) is a subtype of primary open-angle glaucoma characterized by progressive optic nerve damage despite intraocular pressure (IOP) remaining within the normal range. The underlying pathophysiology of NTG remains incompletely understood, and its diagnosis is often delayed due to the lack of a definitive screening tool. This study aimed to evaluate differences in intracranial pressure pulse wave amplitude recorded from closed eyelids between NTG patients and control subjects using a novel non-invasive monitoring technology. *Materials and Methods*: A cross-sectional observational study was conducted, enrolling NTG patients and age-matched controls. Intracranial pressure pulse wave signals were recorded from closed eyelids using the 'Archimedes' 02 device, which employs a highly sensitive digital pressure sensor and hydromechanical coupling for signal transmission. The amplitude of recorded intracranial pressure pulse waves was analyzed and compared between groups. Statistical analyses were performed using IBM SPSS Statistics 30.0, with significance set at $p < 0.05$. *Results*: A total of 140 participants were enrolled, including 68 NTG patients and 72 controls. After applying exclusion criteria, 63 NTG patients and 68 controls were included in the final analysis. The median intracranial pressure pulse wave amplitude was significantly higher in NTG patients (0.1326 a.u.) than in controls (0.0889 a.u.), with $p = 0.01$. *Conclusions*: These findings suggest that intracranial pressure pulse wave monitoring may serve as a potential biomarker for NTG. Further studies are needed to determine the diagnostic accuracy, sensitivity, and specificity of this technology for NTG detection.

Keywords: normal-tension glaucoma; non-invasive monitoring; intracranial pressure pulse waves; glaucoma screening

1. Introduction

Glaucoma is a progressive optic neuropathy involving the degeneration of retinal ganglion cells and damage to the optic nerve head, leading to visual field deterioration and, if left untreated, irreversible blindness [1–3]. Glaucoma is categorized based on its anatomical and pathophysiological characteristics, with open-angle and angle-closure representing the two main subtypes [4]. Differentiating between open-angle and angle-closure glaucoma relies on a thorough evaluation of the anterior chamber angle using gonioscopy [4,5]. Open-angle glaucoma is characterized by a wide angle between the iris and the cornea; however, aqueous humour drainage is impaired, leading to a gradual increase in intraocular pressure (IOP) and the progression of the disease, often without noticeable symptoms [6–8]. In closed-angle glaucoma, the drainage angle between the iris and the cornea becomes closed, commonly due to the iris pushing forward. This usually leads to a rapid increase in IOP and the development of symptoms such as ocular pain, redness, decreased vision, and headaches [6,9]. Glaucoma is also classified as primary or secondary [4,10]. When the disease occurs without an identifiable cause, both open-angle and closed-angle glaucoma are termed primary glaucoma [4]. Secondary glaucoma describes any type of glaucoma caused by an identifiable factor leading to increased IOP and subsequent optic nerve damage [4].

Primary open-angle glaucoma (POAG) is the most common form of glaucoma, with an estimated 52.68 million cases among the adult population aged 40–80 years in 2020 [11]. It is projected that the global prevalence of glaucoma will reach 111.8 million cases by 2040, driven by factors such as population ageing and growth [12].

Normal-tension glaucoma (NTG) is a subtype of primary open-angle glaucoma characterized by glaucomatous optic nerve damage occurring in patients whose IOP consistently remains below 21 mmHg [4,13,14]. The pathogenesis of NTG is poorly understood and remains under investigation. Recent findings suggest that impaired ocular blood flow, an increased translaminar pressure gradient, disrupted cerebrospinal fluid circulation, neurodegenerative disorders, oxidative stress, genetic factors, and abnormal biomechanics of the lamina cribrosa contribute to the etiology of the condition [15–18]. The proportion of NTG among primary open-angle glaucoma cases varies widely, ranging from 30% in an Italian study to as high as 92% in a Japanese investigation, and is influenced by ethnicity [19–21]. However, the proportion of NTG among patients with POAG in glaucoma clinics worldwide is generally less than 30% [21]. These figures highlight global underdiagnosis, letting NTG progress go unchecked and potentially causing blindness [21].

There is a growing demand for innovative screening techniques to enable early glaucoma diagnosis. A group of researchers from Canada has developed a sophisticated Fourier-domain optical coherence tomography system to measure subtle pulsations in ocular structures [22]. In a study with glaucoma patients, they found that the amplitude of pulsatility in ocular elements, such as the axial distance between the retina and the optic disc cup, is significantly greater in glaucoma patients compared to controls [23].

We recently developed a novel, non-invasive method and system for monitoring intracranial pressure waves [24]. This technology captures pulsations as pressure signals through the closed eyelid using a highly sensitive pressure sensor and hydromechanical coupling. To ensure efficient signal transmission from the pulsating outer ocular structures to the digital pressure sensor, two chambers filled with a non-compressible liquid were designed—one for each eye. A thin elastic film acts as a sealing layer to prevent direct contact between the closed eyelid and the fluid. In this study, we aimed to evaluate differences in the amplitude of pressure pulse waves recorded with this technology between patients with normal-tension glaucoma and control subjects.

2. Materials and Methods

2.1. Study Design and Participants

We conducted a cross-sectional observational study in accordance with the STROBE recommendations [25]. The Kaunas Regional Biomedical Research Ethics Committee approved the study (Approval No. BE-2-15, dated 2024-02-10), and it was conducted in compliance with the ethical principles outlined in the Declaration of Helsinki [26]. The study was also registered on ClinicalTrials.gov (Registration No.: NCT06443411).

Normal-tension glaucoma patients and control group subjects were recruited from the Hospital of the Lithuanian University of Health Sciences Kaunas Clinics between 22 April 2024 and 3 February 2025.

Participants in the study group were patients diagnosed with NTG before our study, confirmed by an ophthalmologist based on characteristic glaucomatous changes in the optic nerve head, visual field defects, an open anterior chamber angle, and an intraocular pressure of IOP $\leq$ 21 mmHg on the daily curve at the time of diagnosis, without the use of antiglaucoma medications. At the time of our study, some NTG patients were not receiving antiglaucoma medication, while others had initiated treatment following the confirmation of their diagnosis by an ophthalmologist. Additionally, the IOP on the day of the study examination was $\leq$21 mmHg in all participants, regardless of their antiglaucoma treatment status.

The control group consisted of subjects without glaucoma (i.e., those with normal-appearing optic nerve heads, no retinal nerve fibre layer [RNFL] thinning, and normal visual fields). Participants in the control group also had no acute or chronic uncompensated conditions that could influence study outcomes. Matching between the NTG and control groups was performed based on age and anthropometric parameters.

Exclusion criteria for both groups were as follows:

1. Refusal to participate;
2. Age under 25 or over 85 years;
3. Pregnancy or breastfeeding;
4. Allergy or sensitivity to local anesthetics;
5. Eye diseases that could distort study results;
6. History of orbital or ocular trauma;
7. Previous ocular surgery;
8. Acute or chronic, currently exacerbated respiratory diseases;
9. Decompensated cardiovascular diseases (e.g., a second- or third-degree atrioventricular block or cardiogenic shock);
10. Decompensated diabetes mellitus;
11. History of neurological disorders or mental illnesses.

2.2. Data Collection

Non-invasive monitoring of pressure pulse waves from closed eyelids was conducted using a recently developed technology called 'Archimedes 02', designed to monitor intracranial pressure waves [24]. The device is gently attached to both closed eyelids and secured with a band around the back of the head. The component in contact with the eyelids consists of a thin (50 µm) non-allergenic elastic film, which transmits pulsations from the closed eyelids to a non-compressible liquid. These pulsations are captured by a highly sensitive digital pressure sensor, which is in direct contact with the liquid. The baseline pressure of the liquid was set to 2.5 mmHg in both eyes of each subject before the monitoring session. Figure 1 shows the device placed on both closed eyelids of a control subject, prepared for intracranial pressure pulse wave monitoring. Pressure pulse wave monitoring was conducted for up to 5 min for each participant. The recorded signals were subsequently processed and analyzed using MATLAB (R2024a, MathWorks, Natick, MA, USA) to calculate the amplitude of the pressure pulse waves.

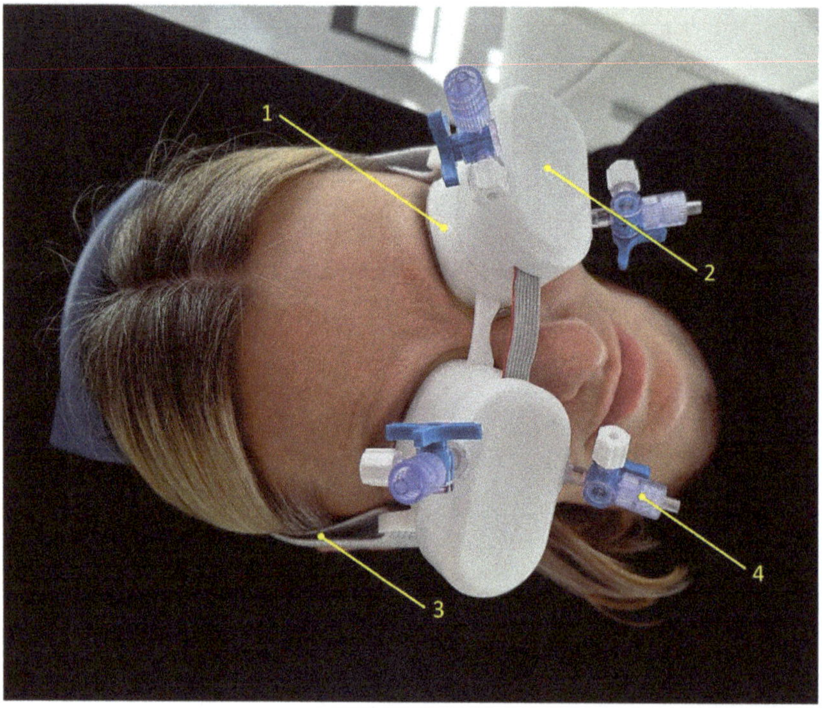

Figure 1. An image of an 'Archimedes 02' monitor placed on both closed eyelids of a control subject. 1—Chamber filled with a non-compressible liquid, 2—sensor assembly containing electronic components and a highly sensitive pressure transducer, 3—headband securing the device to the head, 4—valve for connecting a tube to fill the chamber with liquid and remove air.

On the day of the examination, the study objectives, methods, and procedures were explained to all participants, who then provided written informed consent. All participants were in a supine position during the procedure, and all examinations were conducted during the daytime, between 8:00 a.m. and 7:00 p.m.

2.3. *Statistical Analysis*

Statistical analysis was performed using IBM SPSS Statistics software (version 30.0; IBM Corporation, Armonk, NY, USA). Two parameters—intraocular pressure and the amplitude of pressure pulse waves—were compared between the normal-tension glaucoma and control groups. The comparisons were conducted first by analyzing the right and left eyes separately, and then by including measurements from both eyes together. For the analysis of data from both eyes, a mixed ANOVA using the General Linear Model (GLM) procedure was applied to assess the effects of both between-group factors (control and NTG) and within-subject factors (left and right eyes). The Kolmogorov–Smirnov test was used to examine the data distribution normality. The analysis of the quantitative variables involved calculating the mean and standard deviation (SD), as well as the median and interquartile range (IQR). To compare the groups, Student's *t*-test was used when the data were normally distributed, and the non-parametric Mann–Whitney U test was applied when the data did not follow a normal distribution. The significance level was set at $p < 0.05$.

3. Results

A total of 140 participants were enrolled in the study, comprising 68 NTG patients and 72 control subjects. A complete flow chart of the study is presented in Figure 2.

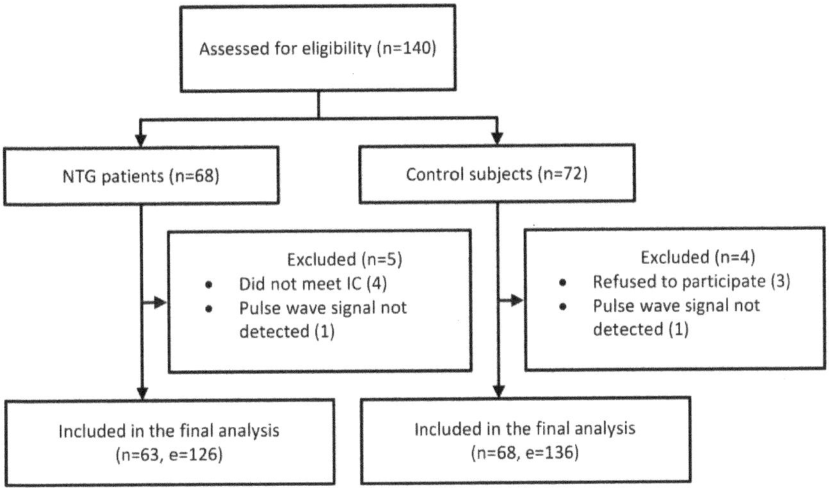

Figure 2. Flow chart of the study. Abbreviations: NTG, normal-tension glaucoma; IC, inclusion criteria; n, number of participants; e, number of eyes.

Following the exclusion, 63 NTG patients and 68 control subjects were included in the statistical analysis. The demographic characteristics of the participants are presented in Table 1, while the medical data are provided in Table 2.

Table 1. Demographic data of the included participants in this comparative study.

Group	Age, Years				Gender			
	Mean	±SD	Min	Max	Male, n	Female, n	Male, %	Female, %
Control	58.91	±12.76	25	84	17	51	25.0	75.0
NTG	66.63	±9.86	43	85	13	50	20.6	79.4

Abbreviations: NTG, normal-tension glaucoma; SD, standard deviation; n, number of participants.

Table 2. Medical data of the participants included in this comparative study.

Group	Control	NTG
NTG medication, n	No medication, 68	No medication, 6 Pg analogues, 47 CAIs, 19 β blockers, 30 α2 agonists, 2

Table 2. *Cont.*

Group	Control	NTG
Comorbidity, n	No comorbidities, 38 Arterial hypertension, 27 Diabetes mellitus, 4 Hypothyroidism, 3 Depression, 2 Gout (podagra), 3 Rheumatoid arthritis, 1 Psoriasis, 1 Asthma, 1 Ischemic heart disease, 3 Gastritis, 1	No comorbidities, 23 Arterial hypertension, 33 Heart failure, 4 Hypercholesterolemia, 4 Parkinson's disease, 1 Autoimmune thyroiditis, 1 Diabetes mellitus, 3 Depression, 1 Gout (podagra), 2 Osteoporosis, 1 Angina pectoris, 2 Chronic atrial fibrillation, 3 BPH, 1 Hyperlipidemia, 1
Systemic medication, n	No systemic medication, 41 CCB, 9 ACE inhibitor, 11 Thyroid hormone, 2 Statin, 10 β-blockers, 13 SSRI, 2 XDH inhibitor, 2 Thiazide-like diuretic, 2 Biguanide, 2 ARB, 3 T4 hormone, 2 Other, 11	No systemic medication, 22 ARB, 6 Thiazide diuretic, 2 Statin, 11 β-blockers, 22 ACE inhibitor, 13 BDZ, 3 NSAID, 6 SIRAs, 2 α2-agonist, 2 Thiazide-like diuretic, 2 XDH inhibitor, 2 Biguanide, 2 CCB, 6 Xa inhibitor, 3 Other, 14

Abbreviations: NTG, normal-tension glaucoma; CS, control subjects; n, number of participants; Pg analogues, prostaglandin analogues; CAIs, carbonic anhydrase inhibitors; BPH, benign prostatic hyperplasia; ARB, angiotensin receptor blocker; ACE inhibitor, angiotensin-converting enzyme inhibitor; BDZ, benzodiazepine; NSAID, non-steroidal anti-inflammatory drug; SIRAs, selective imidazoline receptor agonists; XDH inhibitor, xanthine dehydrogenase inhibitor; CCB, calcium channel blocker; Xa inhibitor, factor Xa inhibitor; SSRI, selective serotonin reuptake inhibitor.

The intraocular pressure data met the assumption of normality, according to the Kolmogorov–Smirnov test, for both groups in each case, with the right and left eyes analyzed separately and then together. The results of Student's *t*-test showed no significant difference in IOP between the groups when comparing the right and left eyes separately. Analysis of IOP data showed no significant interaction between groups and eyes ($F(1, 129) = 2.214$, $p = 0.139$), no significant within-subject effect (left and right eyes; $F(1, 129) = 2.311$, $p = 0.133$), and no significant between-subjects effect (NTG and control groups; $F(1, 129) = 2.242$, $p = 0.137$). The results of the statistical analysis are presented in Table 3, and the boxplots of the IOP measurements are shown in Figure 3.

Table 3. Results of statistical tests for IOP measurements.

Analyzed Eyes	Left		Right		Both	
Group	Control	NTG	Control	NTG	Control	NTG
Mean (±SD)	15.39 (±3.20)	14.80 (±2.78)	15.39 (±3.15)	14.43 (±2.93)	15.39 (±3.16)	14.62 (±2.85)
Median (IQR)	15.15 (13.00–17.22)	14.50 (12.70–17.00)	15.30 (12.70–17.65)	14.70 (12.30–16.70)	15.30 (12.78–17.30)	14.60 (12.70–16.70)
K-S test *p*-value	0.200	0.200	0.200	0.200	0.052	0.200
Significance between groups	t = 1.112, df = 129, $p = 0.268$		t = 1.795, df = 129, $p = 0.075$		$F(1, 129) = 2.242$, $p = 0.137$	

Abbreviations: IOP, intraocular pressure; NTG, normal-tension glaucoma; SD, standard deviation; IQR, interquartile range; K-S test, Kolmogorov–Smirnov test; t, Student's *t*-test statistic; df, degrees of freedom; F, F-statistic from the mixed ANOVA test, used to assess between-subjects effects.

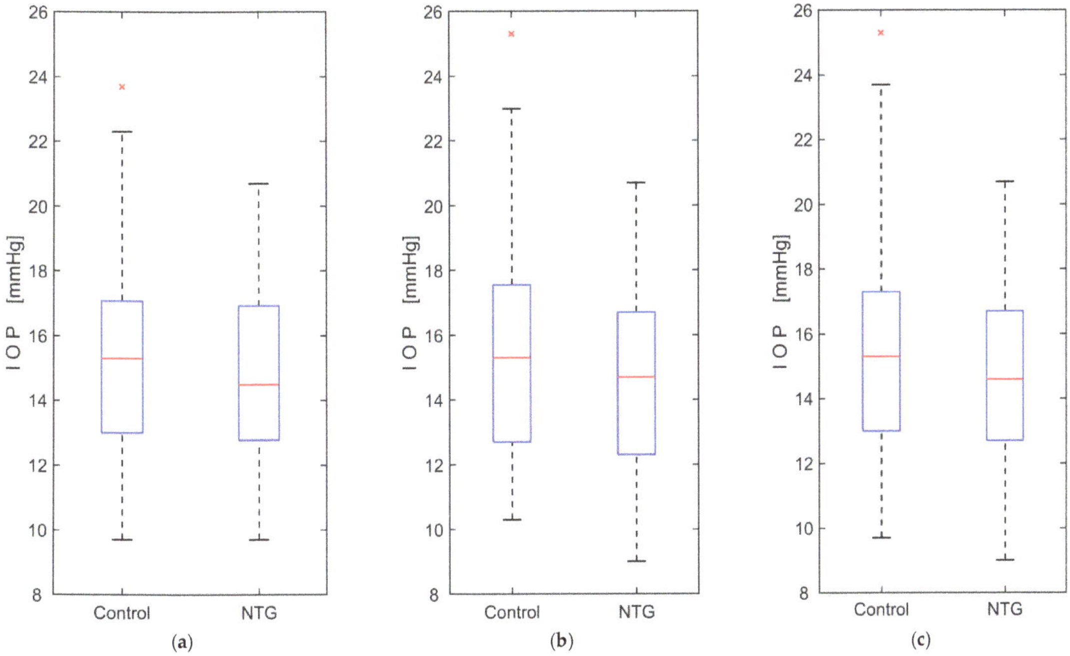

Figure 3. Boxplots of intraocular pressure (IOP) measurements comparing normal-tension glaucoma (NTG) patients and control subjects: (**a**) measurements from the left eye only; (**b**) measurements from the right eye only; (**c**) measurements from both eyes. The red lines represent the medians, while the red crosses (×) indicate statistical outliers.

The registered intracranial pressure pulse wave amplitude data did not meet the assumption of normality, as confirmed by the Kolmogorov–Smirnov test, for both groups in each case, with the right and left eyes were analyzed separately and then combined. A non-parametric Mann–Whitney U test was used to compare the groups and revealed statistically significant differences in amplitude between the NTG and control groups, both when the right and left eyes were compared separately and when both eyes were analyzed together. Analysis of amplitude data showed no significant interaction between groups and eyes ($F(1, 129) = 1.196$, $p = 0.276$), no significant within-subject effect (left and right eyes; $F(1, 129) = 0.001$, $p = 0.978$), but a significant main effect between subjects (NTG and control groups; F(1, 129) = 6.901, $p = 0.01$). The results of the statistical analysis are presented in Table 4, and the boxplots of the amplitude measurements are shown in Figure 4.

Table 4. Results of statistical tests for pulse wave amplitude measurements.

Analyzed Eyes	**Left**		**Right**		**Both**	
Group	Control	NTG	Control	NTG	Control	NTG
Mean (±SD)	0.1106 (±0.0746)	0.1539 (±0.1068)	0.1176 (±0.0771)	0.1466 (±0.0875)	0.1141 (±0.0757)	0.1503 (±0.0973)
Median (IQR)	0.0869 (0.0664–0.1433)	0.1347 (0.0798–0.1967)	0.0921 (0.0659–0.1447)	0.1315 (0.0769–0.1775)	0.0889 (0.0663–0.1434)	0.1326 (0.0769–0.0185)
K-S test p-value	<0.001	0.007	<0.001	0.006	<0.001	<0.001
Significance between groups	U = 1501.0, Z = −2.953, $p = 0.003$		U = 1620.4, Z = −2.402, $p = 0.016$		F(1, 129) = 6.901, $p = 0.01$	

Abbreviations: NTG, normal-tension glaucoma; SD, standard deviation; IQR, interquartile range; K-S test, Kolmogorov–Smirnov test; U, Mann–Whitney test U statistic; Z, Mann–Whitney statistics Z score; F, F-statistic from the mixed ANOVA test, used to assess between-subjects effects.

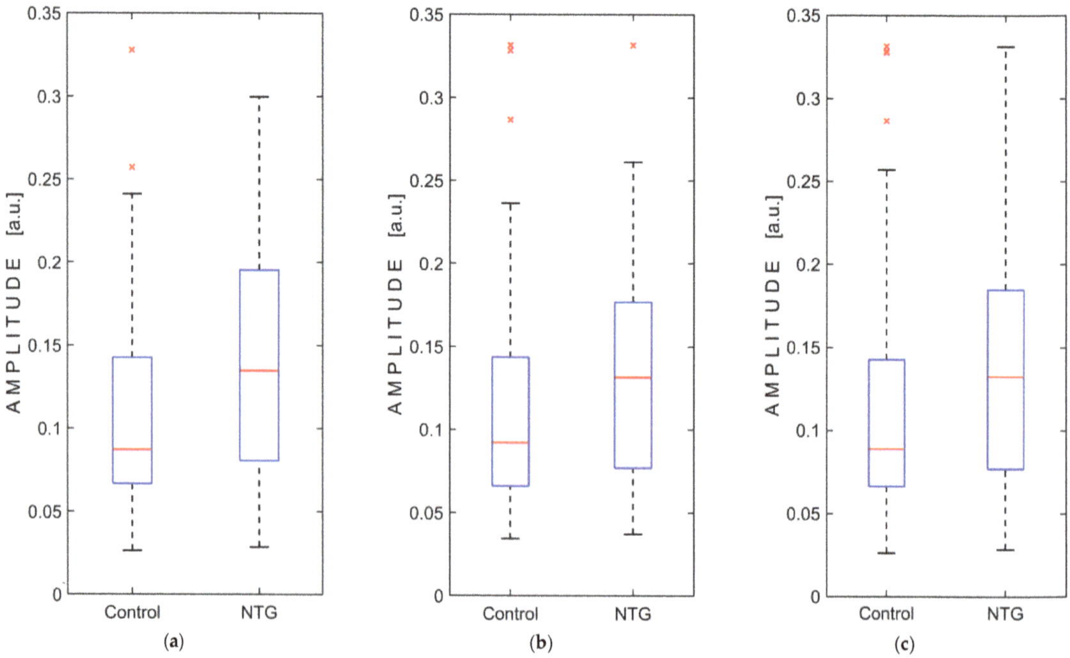

Figure 4. Boxplots of pressure pulse wave amplitude measurements comparing normal-tension glaucoma (NTG) patients and control subjects: (**a**) measurements from the left eye only; (**b**) measurements from the right eye only; (**c**) measurements from both eyes. Abbreviation: a.u., arbitrary units. The red lines represent the medians, while the red crosses (×) indicate statistical outliers.

4. Discussion

Although the condition now termed normal-tension glaucoma was first described in the mid-19th century and its underlying mechanisms have been extensively explored in recent decades, they remain incompletely understood, and the disease continues to be significantly underdiagnosed [15,21,27]. A simple screening tool for evaluating normal-tension glaucoma would be valuable for ophthalmologists.

Researchers led by Singh et al. conducted a study measuring the pulsatile movement of the optic nerve head and the peripapillary retina using a novel Fourier-domain optical coherence tomography system [23]. They found that the mean fundus pulsation amplitude on the nasal side of the optic disc was significantly greater in glaucoma patients compared to normal subjects.

We recently developed non-invasive intracranial pressure wave monitoring technology [24]. This technology is based on the hypothesis that cerebrospinal fluid pulsations in the retrolaminar space along the optic nerve are transmitted to the outer ocular structures, where they can be detected through the closed eyelid as subtle pressure changes. In this paper, we investigated the amplitude of pressure pulse waves recorded from closed eyelids using the 'Archimedes 02' device in patients with normal-tension glaucoma and control subjects.

Subjects diagnosed with NTG by an ophthalmologist prior to our study were recruited for the study group, while the control group consisted of subjects with no history or diagnosis of glaucoma. We found that the mean intraocular pressure, measured in both eyes on the day of the examination, was 14.62 mmHg (SD = $\pm$2.85 mmHg) for the NTG group and 15.39 mmHg (SD = $\pm$3.16 mmHg) for the control group. The observed mean IOP for both groups fell within the normal range of 10–21 mmHg, which is considered typical for healthy subjects and NTG patients with glaucomatous damage [4,28].

This observational study showed a statistically significant difference (p = 0.01) in the amplitude of intracranial pressure pulse waves recorded from both closed eyelids, comparing the NTG group (median amplitude: 0.1326 a.u.) and the control group (median amplitude: 0.0889 a.u.). A statistically significant difference between groups was also observed when the recorded amplitude was analyzed separately, first for the left eye (p = 0.003) and then for the right eye (p = 0.016).

Several limitations of our study are worth mentioning. The gender ratio was skewed, with females comprising 75% of the control group and 79.4% of the NTG group. A larger sample size of male participants is needed to investigate potential differences in pressure pulse wave amplitude between genders. The greater proportion of female subjects enrolled in this study might be explained by findings from other studies indicating that normal-tension glaucoma is more common in women, or by the fact that females tend to live longer than males [14]. Age is epidemiologically considered to be a risk factor for NTG, and the likelihood of developing the disease increases with age [14,29]. The mean age of normal-tension glaucoma patients reported in many studies is in the 60s, which is consistent with the mean age of NTG patients (66 years) observed in this study [14,29]. However, at this age, individuals are often affected by many other health conditions. In this study, both the patients with normal-tension glaucoma and the control group had additional health conditions, such as high blood pressure, diabetes, heart disease, high cholesterol, and others. These conditions were treated with medications that affect the whole body (systemic medications). The influence of specific diseases or medications on the pressure pulse waves recorded using the technology in this study is not yet known.

While the results of this study demonstrate a significant difference in intracranial pressure pulse wave amplitude between NTG patients and controls, it is important to acknowledge that these findings do not yet establish the new measurement method as a replacement for existing clinical practices, such as slit-lamp examinations and tonometry. The 'Archimedes 02' technology shows promise as a potential supplementary tool, but further research and validation are necessary to confirm its clinical utility and diagnostic accuracy. Consequently, its role in routine ophthalmological practice remains exploratory at this stage.

In addition to its potential as a supplementary diagnostic tool, the 'Archimedes 02' technology may offer a foundation for individualized diagnostic support in the future. Although the current experimental results do not allow for its immediate application at the individual level, the ability to reflect personal physiological characteristics presents an intriguing avenue for further investigation. Additional studies involving diverse patient groups are essential to better understand individual differences in measurement results.

The findings of this observational study highlight the need for a prospective clinical investigation into the potential of 'Archimedes 02' as a screening tool for normal-tension glaucoma. Future research should focus on establishing a threshold for pulse wave amplitude to distinguish between healthy individuals and those with NTG. Subsequently, a randomized, double-blinded study involving both controls and NTG patients diagnosed by an ophthalmologist will be essential to assess the diagnostic accuracy, sensitivity, and specificity of 'Archimedes 02'. Such studies will be crucial for determining whether this technology can evolve from a promising concept to a reliable tool of clinical practice.

5. Conclusions

In this study, we demonstrated that non-invasive technology designed to monitor intracranial pressure waves can detect pressure pulse waves through the closed eyelid in normal-tension glaucoma patients, and that these waves have a significantly greater amplitude in NTG patients compared to control subjects. The role of this technology in screening for normal-tension glaucoma needs to be further investigated.

Author Contributions: Conceptualization, L.B. and A.R.; data curation, L.B., S.K., U.K., A.J., A.Z., A.S., E.C. and M.D.; formal analysis, L.B., U.K., E.C., F.S. and K.B.; funding acquisition, S.K. and I.J.; investigation, L.B., S.K., U.K., A.J., A.Z., E.C. and Y.H.; methodology, L.B., S.K., K.B., I.J. and A.R.; project administration, S.K.; resources, U.K., A.J., A.Z., A.S., I.J. and A.R.; software, E.C., M.D. and F.S.; supervision, S.K. and I.J.; validation, L.B., E.C. and K.B.; visualization, L.B. and K.B.; writing—original draft, L.B. and U.K.; writing—review and editing, L.B., S.K., A.S., Y.H., I.J. and A.R. All authors have read and agreed to the published version of the manuscript.

Funding: This research was supported by the Research Council of Lithuania under Grant Agreement No. SV5-40.

Institutional Review Board Statement: This study was conducted in accordance with the Declaration of Helsinki, approved by the Kaunas Regional Biomedical Research Ethics Committee (Approval No. BE-2-15, dated 10 February 2024), and registered in the ClinicalTrials.gov database (Registration No.: NCT06443411).

Informed Consent Statement: Informed consent was obtained from all subjects involved in the study.

Data Availability Statement: Due to privacy concerns and ethical considerations, access to the clinical data used in this study is restricted. The data are available upon reasonable request, subject to approval by the Regional Kaunas Biomedical Research Ethics Committee (kaunorbtek@lsmuni.lt).

Conflicts of Interest: L.B., A.R., E.C., Y.H., and M.D. are the inventors of a non-invasive intracranial pressure pulse wave monitoring technology (US and EU patents pending). This research was supported by the Research Council of Lithuania under Grant Agreement No. SV5-40. L.B., S.K., U.K., A.J., A.Z., F.S., and I.J. received support. The funders had no role in the design of the study; in the collection, analyses, or interpretation of data; in the writing of the manuscript; or in the decision to publish the results.

References

1. Gupta, D.; Chen, P.P. Glaucoma. *Am. Fam. Physician.* **2016**, *93*, 668–674. [PubMed]
2. Allison, K.; Patel, D.; Alabi, O. Epidemiology of Glaucoma: The Past, Present, and Predictions for the Future. *Cureus.* **2020**, *12*, e11686. [CrossRef] [PubMed]
3. Siaudvytyte, L.; Januleviciene, I.; Ragauskas, A.; Bartusis, L.; Meiliuniene, I.; Siesky, B.; Harris, A. The difference in translaminar pressure gradient and neuroretinal rim area in glaucoma and healthy subjects. *J. Ophthalmol.* **2014**, *2014*, 937360. [CrossRef]
4. Harasymowycz, P.; Birt, C.; Gooi, P.; Heckler, L.; Hutnik, C.; Jinapriya, D.; Shuba, L.; Yan, D.; Day, R. MedicaWl Management of Glaucoma in the 21st Century from a Canadian Perspective. *J. Ophthalmol.* **2016**, *2016*, 6509809. [CrossRef]
5. Canadian Ophthalmological Society Glaucoma Clinical Practice Guideline Expert Committee; Canadian Ophthalmological Society. Canadian Ophthalmological Society evidence-based clinical practice guidelines for the management of glaucoma in the adult eye [published correction appears in *Can. J. Ophthalmol.* **2009**, *44*, 477]. *Can. J. Ophthalmol.* **2009**, *44* (Suppl. S1), S7–S93. [CrossRef]
6. Khalil, T.; Khalil, S.; Syed, A.M. Review of Machine Learning techniques for glaucoma detection and prediction. In Proceedings of the 2014 Science and Information Conference, Seoul, Republic of Korea, 6–9 May 2014; pp. 438–442.
7. Srivastava, N.; Chandra, M.; Nitesh. A review exploring the dynamic of aqueous humor and glaucoma: Open & close angle perspective. *Eur. J. Pharm. Med. Res.* **2024**, *11*, 233–248.
8. Johnson, M.; McLaren, J.W.; Overby, D.R. Unconventional aqueous humor outflow: A review. *Exp. Eye Res.* **2017**, *158*, 94–111. [CrossRef]
9. Weinreb, R.N.; Aung, T.; Medeiros, F.A. The pathophysiology and treatment of glaucoma: A review. *JAMA* **2014**, *311*, 1901–1911. [CrossRef]
10. Dietze, J.; Blair, K.; Zeppieri, M.; Havens, S.J. Glaucoma. In *StatPearls [Internet]*; StatPearls Publishing: Treasure Island, FL, USA, 2024. [PubMed]
11. Zhang, N.; Wang, J.; Li, Y.; Jiang, B. Prevalence of primary open angle glaucoma in the last 20 years: A meta-analysis and systematic review. *Sci Rep.* **2021**, *11*, 13762. [CrossRef]
12. Tham, Y.C.; Li, X.; Wong, T.Y.; Quigley, H.A.; Aung, T.; Cheng, C.-Y. Global prevalence of glaucoma and projections of glaucoma burden through 2040: A systematic review and meta-analysis. *Ophthalmology* **2014**, *121*, 2081–2090. [CrossRef]
13. Mroczkowska, S.; Benavente-Perez, A.; Negi, A.; Sung, V.; Patel, S.R.; Gherghel, D. Primary open-angle glaucoma vs normal-tension glaucoma: The vascular perspective. *JAMA Ophthalmol.* **2013**, *131*, 36–43. [CrossRef]
14. Mi, X.S.; Yuan, T.F.; So, K.F. The current research status of normal tension glaucoma. *Clin. Interv. Aging* **2014**, *9*, 1563–1571. [CrossRef] [PubMed]
15. Killer, H.E.; Pircher, A. Normal tension glaucoma: Review of current understanding and mechanisms of the pathogenesis. *Eye* **2018**, *32*, 924–930. [CrossRef]
16. Adeghate, J.; Rahmatnejad, K.; Waisbourd, M.; Katz, L.J. Intraocular pressure-independent management of normal tension glaucoma. *Surv. Ophthalmol.* **2019**, *64*, 101–110. [CrossRef] [PubMed]
17. Wiggs, J.L.; Pasquale, L.R. Genetics of glaucoma. *Hum. Mol. Genet.* **2017**, *26*, R21–R27. [CrossRef] [PubMed]
18. Chen, M.J. Normal tension glaucoma in Asia: Epidemiology, pathogenesis, diagnosis, and management. *Taiwan J. Ophthalmol.* **2020**, *10*, 250–254. [CrossRef]
19. Bonomi, L.; Marchini, G.; Marraffa, M.; Bernardi, P.; De Franco, I.; Perfetti, S.; Varotto, A.; Tenna, V. Prevalence of glaucoma and intraocular pressure distribution in a defined population. The Egna-Neumarkt Study. *Ophthalmology* **1998**, *105*, 209–215. [CrossRef]
20. Iwase, A.; Suzuki, Y.; Araie, M.; Yamamoto, T.; Abe, H.; Shirato, S.; Kuwayama, Y.; Mishima, H.K.; Shimizu, H.; Tomita, G.; et al. The prevalence of primary open-angle glaucoma in Japanese: The Tajimi Study. *Ophthalmology* **2004**, *111*, 1641–1648. [CrossRef]
21. Lee, J.W.Y.; Chan, P.P.; Zhang, X.; Chen, L.J.; Jonas, J.B. Latest Developments in Normal-Pressure Glaucoma: Diagnosis, Epidemiology, Genetics, Etiology, Causes and Mechanisms to Management. *Asia Pac. J. Ophthalmol.* **2019**, *8*, 457–468. [CrossRef]
22. Singh, K.; Dion, C.; Wajszilber, M.; Ozaki, T.; Lesk, M.R.; Costantino, S. Measurement of ocular fundus pulsation in healthy subjects using a novel Fourier-domain optical coherence tomography. *Invest. Ophthalmol. Vis. Sci.* **2011**, *52*, 8927–8932. [CrossRef]
23. Singh, K.; Dion, C.; Godin, A.G.; Lorghaba, F.; Descovich, D.; Wajszilber, M.; Ozaki, T.; Costantino, S.; Lesk, M.R. Pulsatile movement of the optic nerve head and the peripapillary retina in normal subjects and in glaucoma. *Invest. Ophthalmol. Vis. Sci.* **2012**, *53*, 7819–7824. [CrossRef] [PubMed]
24. Putnynaite, V.; Chaleckas, E.; Deimantavicius, M.; Bartusis, L.; Hamarat, Y.; Petkus, V.; Karaliunas, A.; Ragauskas, A. Prospective comparative clinical trials of novel non-invasive intracranial pressure pulse wave monitoring technologies: Preliminary clinical data. *Interface Focus.* **2024**, *14*, 20240027. [CrossRef]
25. von Elm, E.; Altman, D.G.; Egger, M.; Pocock, S.J.; Gotzsche, P.C.; Vandenbroucke, J.P. Strengthening the Reporting of Observational Studies in Epidemiology (STROBE) statement: Guidelines for reporting observational studies. *BMJ* **2007**, *335*, 806–808. [CrossRef] [PubMed]

26. World Medical Association. World Medical Association Declaration of Helsinki: Ethical Principles for Medical Research Involving Human Participants. *JAMA* **2025**, *333*, 71–74. [CrossRef]
27. Trivli, A.; Koliarakis, I.; Terzidou, C.; Siganos, C.S.; Dalianis, G.; Detorakis, E.T.; Goulielmos, G.N.; Spandidos, D.A. Normal-tension glaucoma: Pathogenesis and genetics. *Exp. Ther. Med.* **2019**, *17*, 563–574. [CrossRef] [PubMed]
28. Wang, Y.X.; Xu, L.; Wei, W.B.; Jonas, J.B. Intraocular pressure and its normal range adjusted for ocular and systemic parameters. The Beijing Eye Study 2011. *PLoS ONE* **2018**, *13*, e0196926. [CrossRef]
29. Lauwers, A.; Barbosa Breda, J.; Stalmans, I. The natural history of untreated ocular hypertension and glaucoma. *Surv. Ophthalmol.* **2023**, *68*, 388–424. [CrossRef]

medicina

MDPI

Review

Ophthalmologic Manifestations in Bardet–Biedl Syndrome: Emerging Therapeutic Approaches

Amaris Rosado [1,*], Ediel Rodriguez [1] and Natalio Izquierdo [2]

[1] School of Medicine, Medical Sciences Campus, University of Puerto Rico, San Juan 00936-5067, Puerto Rico; ediel.rodriguez@upr.edu
[2] Department of Ophthalmology, Medical Sciences Campus, University of Puerto Rico, San Juan 00936-5067, Puerto Rico; njuan@msn.com
* Correspondence: amaris.rosado@upr.edu

Abstract: Bardet–Biedl syndrome (BBS) is a rare multisystem ciliopathy characterized by early-onset retinal degeneration and other vision-threatening ophthalmologic manifestations. This review synthesizes current knowledge on the ocular phenotype of BBS as well as emerging therapeutic approaches aimed at preserving visual function. Retinal degeneration, particularly early macular involvement and rod–cone dystrophy, remains the hallmark of BBS-related vision loss. Additional ocular manifestations, such as refractive errors, nystagmus, optic nerve abnormalities, and cataracts further contribute to visual morbidity. Experimental therapies—including gene-based interventions and pharmacologic strategies such as nonsense suppression and antioxidant approaches—have shown promise in preclinical models but require further validation. Early ophthalmologic care, including routine visual assessments, refractive correction, and low-vision rehabilitation, remains the standard of management. However, there are currently no effective therapies to halt or reverse retinal degeneration, which underscores the importance of emerging molecular and genetic interventions. Timely recognition and comprehensive ophthalmologic evaluation are essential to mitigate visual decline in BBS. Future efforts should focus on translating these approaches into clinical practice, enhancing early diagnosis, and promoting multidisciplinary collaboration to improve long-term outcomes for patients with BBS.

Keywords: Bardet–Biedl syndrome; retinal degeneration; rod–cone dystrophy; ciliopathy; photoreceptor degeneration; gene therapy

1. Introduction

Ciliopathies are a group of disorders caused by impaired function of the primary cilium, resulting in a wide spectrum of clinical manifestations. Cilia are broadly classified into two types: motile and non-motile (primary). Motile cilia are mainly involved in fluid transport, cell motility, and clearing particles across epithelial surfaces. In contrast, primary cilia function as sensory organelles that mediate intracellular signaling essential for normal tissue development and homeostasis [1,2]. These cilia regulate key signaling pathways such as Hedgehog, Wnt, Notch, and mTOR, which are critical for cell polarity, differentiation, and proliferation [3,4]. Dysfunction of primary cilia can lead to isolated organ disease or complex multisystem syndromes, such as BBS, which may include retinal degeneration, renal anomalies, polydactyly, and obesity [5].

BBS is a rare inherited disorder classified as a primary ciliopathy. It is caused by autosomal recessive mutations in genes critical for ciliary structure and function. To date,

27 genes have been identified as causative, most of which encode components of the BBSome complex, chaperonin-like proteins, or elements involved in intraflagellar transport (IFT) [6,7]. The most frequently implicated genes are BBS1 and BBS10, accounting for the majority of molecularly confirmed cases [8,9].

The incidence of BBS is estimated to be between 1 in 120,000 and 160,000 in the United States and Europe, with significantly higher rates reported in genetically isolated populations [8,9]. Due to its genetic pleiotropy and high heterogeneity, BBS presents with a wide range of phenotypic features. Diagnosis is typically based on the presence of either four major features or three major plus two minor features [10]. Major manifestations include rod–cone dystrophy, truncal obesity, postaxial polydactyly, cognitive impairment, learning difficulties, hypogonadism, renal anomalies, and genitourinary abnormalities. Minor features consist of diabetes mellitus, ataxia, hypertonia, oral and dental abnormalities, congenital heart defects, hepatic fibrosis, facial dysmorphism, digital anomalies such as syndactyly, and impaired olfaction [6].

As with other syndromic ciliopathies, the most common and consistent feature in BBS is retinal rod–cone dystrophy, which affects both peripheral and central vision [11,12]. Despite its early onset, the diagnosis of BBS is frequently delayed and often made only after ophthalmologic evaluation [6]. In many cases, symptoms of retinal dystrophy, such as night blindness (nyctalopia), hyperopic astigmatism, ptosis, or mild blepharospasm during early childhood are the initial reasons for seeking medical care [8,13,14]. The condition progresses slowly but often worsens substantially by the second and third decades of life, leading to severe visual impairment or legal blindness [6,13]. Currently, there is no effective therapy to prevent or reverse the retinal degeneration associated with BBS [4,8].

Despite increasing recognition of BBS as a syndromic ciliopathy, the full ophthalmologic spectrum remains insufficiently defined. Most clinical reports focus narrowly on rod–cone dystrophy, often neglecting the broader constellation of ocular abnormalities—including refractive errors, strabismus, nystagmus, optic disc pallor, early cataracts, glaucoma, and macular edema—that significantly impact long-term visual outcomes [8,13,15].

This review addresses these gaps by providing an updated and integrative synthesis of both major and minor ophthalmologic manifestations, while also highlighting recent advances in experimental therapies that may inform future clinical translation. By integrating molecular mechanisms, clinical phenotypes, and translational innovations, we aim to support precision medicine approaches and guide future research priorities in syndromic retinal disease.

2. Methodology

This review followed a structured literature search to synthesize current knowledge on the ophthalmologic manifestations of BBS and emerging therapeutic approaches. The process involved defining the research scope, performing database searches, applying inclusion/exclusion criteria, and organizing the findings thematically. AI-powered tools including EndNote, Grammarly, ChatGPT, Open Evidence, and Perplexity were used to assist with the literature management, thematic synthesis, citation tracking, and language editing.

2.1. Database Selection and Search Strategy

Peer-reviewed articles and publicly available clinical trial records were identified using PubMed, Scopus, Web of Science, Google Scholar, and official clinical trial registries (e.g., ClinicalTrials.gov). The literature search was limited to studies published between January 1995 and May 2024, and only English-language articles were included in the final synthesis. The literature search was conducted using Boolean operators (AND, OR) and included combinations of terms such as "Bardet–Biedl Syndrome," "retinal degeneration," "rod–cone dystrophy," "ocular manifestations," "gene therapy," "ciliopathy," "CRISPR", and "neuroprotective treatment." Relevant studies describing ophthalmologic manifestations or therapeutic strategies for BBS were prioritized.

2.2. Inclusion and Exclusion Criteria

Inclusion criteria were defined to ensure that selected studies were relevant and of high academic quality. Articles were included if they met the criteria below:

- Focused on ophthalmologic findings in patients with molecularly or clinically confirmed BBS;
- Addressed genotype–phenotype correlations or underlying genetic mechanisms relevant to ocular pathology in BBS;
- Described therapeutic interventions targeting visual outcomes in BBS.

Studies were excluded if they met the criteria below:

- Did not specifically address ophthalmologic manifestations or therapeutic approaches related to visual outcomes in BBS;
- Lacked clinical applicability or focused exclusively on non-ocular systemic features of BBS.

2.3. Data Extraction and Thematic Synthesis

Eligible articles were reviewed for relevant information on ocular phenotypes, disease progression, genotype associations, and therapeutic interventions. To minimize bias, two independent reviewers conducted the screening and data extraction process in duplicate, with discrepancies resolved through discussion and consensus. Findings were grouped into thematic categories: (1) retinal pathology and photoreceptor dysfunction; (2) additional ocular features; (3) emerging therapies targeting visual outcomes; and (4) current standards for ophthalmologic evaluation and management in BBS. AI tools were used to facilitate reference management and synthesis. The final manuscript integrates both molecular and clinical perspectives to provide a comprehensive overview of visual pathology and treatment advances in BBS.

3. Pathogenesis, Pathophysiology, and Genetics of Bardet–Biedl Syndrome

Retinal dystrophy is the most consistent and vision-limiting manifestation of BBS, arising from fundamental defects in ciliary structure and function that disrupt photoreceptor maintenance and survival [8,16,17]. In photoreceptor cells, the primary cilium forms the connecting bridge between the inner segment (IS) and outer segment (OS), acting as a specialized conduit for the bidirectional transport of phototransduction proteins from their site of synthesis in the IS to their functional location in the OS [8,16].

BBS genes are directly involved in cilium biogenesis and function, with BBS1 and BBS10 being the most frequently mutated in affected patients [17]. Seven core BBS proteins (BBS1, 2, 4, 5, 7, 8, and 9) form the BBSome complex, which mediates vesicular trafficking to the ciliary membrane, while a chaperonin-like complex composed of BBS6 (MKKS), BBS10, and BBS12 facilitates its assembly [18]. The BBSome cooperates with the IFT system to ensure proper delivery and turnover of phototransduction proteins within the cilium [19,20]. Mutations in these genes disrupt trafficking, leading to protein mislocalization, ciliary congestion, oxidative stress, and ultimately, apoptotic photoreceptor death [21]. In addition to impairing protein trafficking, BBS-related ciliary dysfunction also disrupts major cellular signaling pathways regulated by the primary cilium, such as Hedgehog, Wnt, Notch, and mTOR, which may contribute to photoreceptor degeneration and broader ocular abnormalities [3,4,16,21].

Histopathologic and ultrastructural studies confirm that the connecting cilium functions as a selective gate, and its disruption results in the accumulation of phototransduction proteins or exclusion of non-resident proteins, culminating in OS disorganization and retinal degeneration [16,20]. Clinically, this manifests as a rod–cone dystrophy, where rod photoreceptors are affected early, followed by progressive cone loss affecting central acuity and color discrimination [17].

While the exact roles of BBS proteins in photoreceptor cells are still not completely understood, several studies have started to shed light on how different gene mutations may lead to retinal degeneration. Mutations in BBSome components (e.g., BBS1 and BBS4) impair the directional transport of key ciliary membrane proteins such as rhodopsin and syntaxin-3, resulting in their abnormal accumulation in the IS and a reduced number in the OS [22]. This disrupts protein polarity and contributes to photoreceptor instability.

A study conducted in BBS1-deficient zebrafish revealed that *BBS1* loss destabilizes the BBSome and leads to accumulation of membrane-associated proteins in the OS, particularly those involved in lipid homeostasis [22]. These alterations are accompanied by elevated unesterified cholesterol levels in the OS and precede morphological abnormalities and functional visual deficits, suggesting a role for *BBS1* in maintaining OS membrane integrity [22]. Further, knock-out studies in BBS5−/− mice showed a complete loss of cone function and mislocalization of cone-specific proteins such as M- and S-opsins, arrestin-4, CNGA3, and GNAT2, highlighting that *BBS5* is essential for subtype-specific protein trafficking and cone photoreceptor survival [23,24].

The severity and timing of degeneration also vary by genotype: patients with the *BBS10* mutation typically develop earlier-onset and more rapid decline compared to those with the *BBS1* mutation, as shown in both clinical and experimental models [25,26]. In *BBS10* knock-out mice, cone electroretinography (ERG) responses are absent by postnatal day 30, and rod responses decline rapidly, resulting in near-complete visual loss by nine months [26]. Structural studies in these mice have demonstrated early OS disorganization and mislocalization of cone proteins such as GNAT2 and OPN1MW by postnatal day 15 [26]. These genotype–phenotype correlations have important clinical implications as patients with *BBS10* mutations tend to experience more rapid visual decline, whereas those with *BBS1* mutations often exhibit milder and later-onset disease, supporting the utility of genetic stratification in prognostic counseling and individualized ophthalmologic surveillance.

Genotype–phenotype correlations also suggest that mutations affecting the chaperonin complex (e.g., *BBS10* and *BBS12*) result in more severe retinal phenotypes due to failure to form the BBSome complex altogether [18]. For instance, experimental models of *BBS10* and *BBS12* loss demonstrate upregulation of endoplasmic reticulum stress markers, sustained activation of the unfolded protein response, and early apoptosis of photoreceptors mediated by caspase-12 [18]. In contrast, mutations in BBSome components (e.g., BBS1, BBS4, and BBS5) allow for partial BBSome complex formation but impair its function. Notably, some BBSome components may have disproportionately critical roles, with mutations in *BBS3* and *BBS8* leading to more severe degeneration than *BBS2* or *BBS5* in murine models [21]. Although rod–cone dystrophy remains the hallmark of BBS-related retinal disease, these findings underscore that other ocular features—such as optic nerve pallor, strabismus, nystagmus, and high refractive errors—likely arise from broader defects in ciliary signaling during eye development and neuro-ocular integration [17,20].

4. Ophthalmologic Manifestations

4.1. Retinal Degeneration

Retinal degeneration is the earliest and most consistent feature of patients with BBS, affecting nearly all individuals diagnosed with the condition [17]. BBS is recognized as the second most common syndromic inherited retinal disease after Usher syndrome [17]. The characteristic degeneration closely resembles a rod–cone pattern as seen in retinitis pigmentosa (RP), where rod photoreceptors degenerate first, followed by cone loss [27,28]. Patients typically present in childhood with nyctalopia and progressive peripheral visual field constriction [29,30]. However, unlike many isolated RP cases, early involvement of the macula is common in BBS, leading to concurrent central vision loss and reduced visual acuity at a young age [11,28]. This early cone-rich macular involvement significantly impairs central vision early in the disease course [12,28]. This characteristic macular involvement has important clinical implications as it supports the need for routine macular assessment in pediatric BBS patients and the early initiation of low-vision rehabilitation to preserve functional vision and optimize developmental outcomes [11,28,29].

Ophthalmoscopic findings in the early stages often reveal a salt-and-pepper pigmentary retinopathy. As the disease progresses, optic disc pallor, attenuation of the retinal vessels, and pigment clumping with bone–spicule pigmentation develop [11,12]. Notably, the macula is affected early in BBS: subtle foveal retinal pigment epithelium mottling or a bull's-eye maculopathy may be evident [31,32]. One retrospective study that investigated the retinal features of 46 patients with BBS revealed that 95% exhibit markedly attenuated arterioles, 84% show diffuse pigmentary retinal alterations, and 55% display bone spicule pigmentation in the mid-periphery [32]. Electroretinography (ERG) in patients with this syndrome typically demonstrates markedly reduced or extinguished rod responses in early childhood, with progressive cone dysfunction, resulting in a flat ERG by the second decade of life [30,33]. These changes correlate clinically with profound visual impairment; the majority of patients with BBS are legally blind by adulthood [29,30].

Although retinal degeneration is a hallmark across all genotypes of BBS, several studies have described genotype–phenotype correlations that may help clinicians predict prognosis. For instance, patients with mutations in BBS1, the most common genotype, have a milder disease course, with a later onset of symptoms and slower decline in visual acuity compared to other subtypes [11,12]. By contrast, patients with mutations in BBS10 have an earlier onset of nyctalopia, more severe reductions in the visual field, and an earlier loss of ERG responses—often by mid-childhood [11,12]. A comparative study of patients with mutations in BBS1 and BBS10 confirmed that ERG abnormalities and a loss of measurable retinal function occur significantly earlier in patients with the mutation in BBS10 [12], supporting a genotype-specific pattern of progression.

Nonetheless, there is considerable clinical heterogeneity, even among individuals carrying identical pathogenic variants. Patients with the same BBS gene mutation may display divergent patterns of central and peripheral vision loss, suggesting the influence of modifier genes, environmental exposures, or epigenetic factors [28,34]. This heterogeneity may also be influenced by triallelic inheritance patterns, where mutations at a second BBS locus can modify the phenotypic expression of a primary biallelic mutation [35]. For example, studies have shown that the presence of a third mutant allele in BBS6 or BBS2 may worsen the clinical phenotype in patients with primary BBS1 mutations, supporting an oligogenic model of inheritance in BBS [35]. Emerging research suggests that environmental exposures, epigenetic modifications, and the presence of modifier genes may partially explain the heterogeneity in visual outcomes observed among patients with identical BBS mutations, highlighting the need for personalized ophthalmologic surveillance and prognostic counseling [28,34]. In other words, although genotype may provide insight into disease severity, it is not a definitive predictor of visual prognosis, and close, individualized ophthalmologic surveillance remains essential regardless of genetic background [11,28].

4.2. Refractive Errors and Corneal Abnormalities

Accumulating evidence supports that the primary cilium plays a critical role in corneal development and maintenance. It regulates signaling pathways essential for epithelial stratification, stromal organization, and corneal transparency during morphogenesis [36]. Moreover, ciliary dysfunction has been implicated in the pathogenesis of corneal disease, including curvature abnormalities and altered corneal homeostasis findings that are particularly relevant in ciliopathies such as BBS [36].

A cross-sectional, retrospective study involving 45 patients with genetically confirmed BBS (mean age 16 years) measured spherical and cylindrical refractive errors and corneal curvature [37]. The study demonstrated a strong association between the syndrome and high corneal astigmatism, with a mean astigmatism of 3.7 ± 1.0 diopters (D) and over half of the cohort exhibiting ≥ 3 D, exceeding the threshold for clinically significant astigmatism [37].

In addition to astigmatism, myopia, hyperopia, and even emmetropia have all been reported among patients with BBS, underscoring the spectrum of refractive profiles. Importantly, several studies have identified genotype–phenotype correlations in refractive outcomes. For example, individuals with BBS1 mutations exhibited a mix of myopia and hyperopia, while those with BBS10 mutations were predominantly myopic with significantly higher rates of myopia compared to BBS1 [38]. Genotypic influences have also been noted in patients with mutations in BBS3 and BBS4, further supporting the role of genetic variation in shaping ocular phenotypes in patients with BBS [39].

Astigmatism was frequently observed across genotypic subgroups and often exceeded 2.0 D, reinforcing its role as a clinically relevant feature of BBS-associated ocular pathology [38]. Given the underlying retinal dysfunction that characterizes BBS, most notably rod–cone dystrophy, early correction of refractive errors is essential. Spectacles or contact lenses should be prescribed promptly to maximize residual visual acuity, particularly in pediatric patients at risk for amblyopia or irreversible visual decline. Although randomized trials in BBS are lacking, retrospective studies and expert consensus support early and aggressive correction of refractive errors—particularly in children—as a strategy to delay amblyopia and maximize visual development during the critical period of cortical plasticity [37,40].

4.3. Strabismus (Ocular Misalignment)

Strabismus has also been described as an ophthalmic finding in patients diagnosed with this syndrome [41,42]. One cohort study found a 26% prevalence of strabismus and nystagmus in patients with BBS [41]. The same study reported that strabismus in these patients manifested as an even distribution between esotropias (inward turning) and exotropias (outward turning) [41]. Nonetheless, another study focusing on pediatric patients with BBS found that approximately 38% had some form of strabismus present at the initial ophthalmologic evaluation [42]—the study noted the greater prevalence of exotropia over esotropia. Due to early vision loss, strabismus in patients with this syndrome has been described as sensory in origin [40].

4.4. Nystagmus

Approximately 10% of patients with BBS have nystagmus, particularly those with early, profound retinal degeneration and severe visual dysfunction [40,43]. However, recent studies suggest a higher prevalence; Milibari and co-workers reported that 37% of patients with BBS presented with nystagmus as an initial ophthalmologic sign [14].

A genotype–phenotype correlation has also been described, with higher rates observed among those carrying severe variants. In a German cohort, 70% of patients with mutations in *BBS10* have nystagmus compared to 27% of those with mutations in *BBS1* [44]. Clinically, nystagmus often appears in early childhood and is typically accompanied by other visual disturbances such as night blindness, photophobia, and peripheral visual field loss [45]. Thus, the presence of early-onset nystagmus in a child with syndromic features should prompt evaluation for BBS as it may reflect significant retinal dysfunction requiring genetic and ophthalmologic assessment [40].

4.5. Cataracts

Cataracts are another ocular complication that have been well described in the literature in patients with BBS [46,47]. It has been described that cataracts tend to develop in patients with BBS during early adulthood [46,47]. Additionally, one study showed that genetic variability may influence the age at which cataracts appear, with a mean age of presentation of 18 years in patients with mutations in *BBS10* compared to 27 years in patients with mutations in *BBS1* [46]. Nasser and co-workers reported that 52% of patients with BBS had cataracts, and many required cataract surgeries to improve visual acuity [44]. In contrast, one pediatric-centered case series described cataracts in only a minority of patients, suggesting that cataract development in BBS may correlate with age and progression of retinal degeneration [48].

4.6. Optic Nerve Abnormalities

Optic nerve abnormalities are a frequently reported ophthalmologic feature in BBS, often characterized by optic disc pallor, atrophy, and narrowing of the retinal arterioles, particularly as the retinal degeneration progresses. These changes are frequently observed during ophthalmoscopic evaluation and are associated with significant visual impairment. These have been consistently reported in patients with the syndrome having advanced stages of retinal disease [17].

A recent German cohort study described that most patients with mutations in *BBS1* and *BBS10* had pale optic discs and macular atrophy [44]. Traditionally, these optic nerve findings have been considered secondary to the outer retinal degeneration; however, some evidence suggests that primary optic neuropathy may also occur. In a study by Iannaccone and co-workers, patients with BBS had early optic disc pallor in the presence of structurally preserved maculae, indicating that optic nerve atrophy may, in certain cases, represent a primary manifestation rather than a downstream consequence of photoreceptor degeneration [49]. Supporting this, advanced spectral-domain optical coherence tomography (SD-OCT) has demonstrated retinal nerve fiber layer (RNFL) thinning, while corneal confocal microscopy has revealed a loss of corneal nerve fibers in patients with BBS—findings that extend beyond photoreceptor involvement and suggest broader neuro-ophthalmologic compromise [50]. Advanced imaging modalities—particularly spectral-domain optical coherence tomography (SD-OCT) and retinal nerve fiber layer (RNFL) analysis—are increasingly recommended in clinical practice to detect early neuro-ophthalmic compromise and to guide longitudinal monitoring in patients with BBS [49,50]. Additionally, although uncommon, structural anomalies such as optic disc drusen and chorioretinal colobomas have been reported in the literature [51,52].

5. Emerging Therapeutic Approaches for Ophthalmologic Complications of BBS

5.1. Gene Therapy

As stated by the American Society of Gene and Cell Therapy, gene therapy is an excellent method to treat and prevent diseases [53]. This therapy targets the underlying genetic cause of a disease through the delivery of genetic material, in the form of DNA or RNA, to alter how a protein is produced by a cell [53]. This new genetic material that is incorporated into the cell can be delivered through a vector, often viruses, that can be administered either ex vivo or in vivo [53]. Ex vivo gene therapy involves removing cells from the patient, modifying them outside the body, and then reintroducing them into the patient [53]. In contrast, in vivo gene therapy involves directly delivering the genetic material into the patient's body, often through injection [53].

Gene therapy offers a promising approach to addressing the genetic defects causing photoreceptor dysfunction and degeneration in the retina of patients with this syndrome. Early proof-of-concept studies have demonstrated that gene augmentation could effectively target retinal degeneration in BBS animal models. A 2011 study showed that subretinal delivery of the *BBS4* gene via an adeno-associated virus (AAV) in *BBS4*-null mice corrected rhodopsin mislocalization, improved photoreceptor outer segment structure, and preserved rod function as confirmed by electroretinogram analysis [54]. Another impactful study was published in 2013, using a knock-in mouse model carrying the common M390R mutation in the *BBS1* gene [55]. Researchers delivered the wild-type *BBS1* gene via an AAV vector through subretinal injection. This intervention partially restored BBS1 protein expression, corrected mislocalized phototransduction proteins, and preserved retinal architecture, resulting in modest but meaningful functional improvements [55].

This 2013 study also revealed a key challenge of gene therapy in patients with BBS—the potential dose-dependent toxicity that the BBS1 protein may cause. Wild-type mice (with no BBS1 deficiency) treated with the wild-type *BBS1* gene developed retinal degeneration [55]. These findings highlight the need to control transgene expression levels to avoid potential overexpression toxicity. In addition to dose-dependent toxicity, translational barriers include immune responses to AAV capsid proteins and the potential for intraocular inflammation following subretinal delivery, which could limit treatment efficacy or preclude redosing [16]. Furthermore, long-term safety remains a critical concern as persistent expression of the transgene may lead to delayed adverse effects, necessitating extended follow-up periods in future clinical trials [16,55,56]. A recent review from the Strasbourg IGMA/CIMERA group, led by H. Dollfus, elaborates on this dose-optimization challenge and details their translational AAV-BBS1 process aimed at mitigating overexpression risks [16].

More recently, a preclinical study focused on *BBS10*, a gene responsible for approximately 21% of cases, has further advanced the field of gene therapy in BBS [57]. In this study, a viral construct carrying the wild-type *BBS10* sequence was delivered subretinally in mouse models to treat retinal degeneration. Results showed that the therapy slowed photoreceptor cell death, preserved retinal structure, and delayed vision loss in the treated eyes. Importantly, cone photoreceptors, which are typically non-functional early in BBS10-related disease, regained measurable electrical function following treatment [57]. These findings are particularly encouraging as they suggest gene therapy could not only halt but also partially reverse cone dysfunction if administered early. The study also reported improvements in visually guided behavior, indicating that gene therapy preserved meaningful visual capacity over time.

Recently, a naturally-occurring *BBS7* mutation was identified in a colony of rhesus macaques, making it the first non-human primate model of BBS [58]. These monkeys exhibited classical BBS features, including progressive retinal degeneration, which Dr. Martha Neuringer and co-workers are currently testing with a subretinal gene therapy [59]. Treated eyes showed slowed degeneration and improved cone-mediated function compared to untreated eyes [59]. Building upon these preclinical successes, the first human clinical trial targeting retinal degeneration in BBS is currently in development; AXV-101 is an investigational gene therapy designed specifically for patients with the missense *BBS1* M390R mutation, the most common genetic cause of BBS [60]. This therapy uses an AAV9 vector to deliver a codon-optimized *BBS1* gene directly to the subretinal space, aiming to preserve photoreceptor cells and slow retinal degeneration. Preclinical studies have demonstrated that AXV-101 halts photoreceptor and outer nuclear retinal layer degeneration in a dose-dependent manner in BBS1M390R animal models. This therapy has shown efficacy and safety; therefore, it is expected to enter clinical trials in 2025 [60]. In addition to AXV-101, preclinical efforts are underway to develop gene therapy vectors for other common subtypes, such as BBS10 and BBS4, although clinical trials have not yet been initiated [52]. Furthermore, alternative delivery approaches, including intravitreal injection, are being explored in other inherited retinal diseases and may offer less invasive options for broader patient access in the future, although subretinal injection remains the preferred route for photoreceptor targeting in BBS at present [56,57,61].

5.2. Gene-Editing Therapies

CRISPR-Cas9 is a powerful gene-editing technology derived from a bacterial immune system that enables targeted modifications to DNA with high precision [62]. It uses a guide RNA to direct the Cas9 nuclease to a specific sequence in the genome, where it creates a double-strand break, allowing the DNA to be disrupted, deleted, or corrected through cellular repair mechanisms [63]. This method has revolutionized molecular biology by enabling researchers to edit genes in living organisms with relative ease, and it holds great promise for treating genetic diseases, including inherited retinal disorders like BBS [64].

Gene-editing therapies such as CRISPR/Cas9 are, therefore, being actively studied to correct the diverse pathogenic variants identified across more than 21 BBS genes [56]. Molinari, Ahmad, and co-workers state that the eye is an ideal organ for in vivo editing because of its surgical accessibility and compartmentalized immune system [61,65]. Further, Kenny and co-workers further emphasize subretinal delivery as a practical first target by keeping the gene-editing machinery confined to the eye and limiting unwanted editing elsewhere in the body [56]. Additionally, this therapy's effect is easy to measure because any benefit or harm can be tracked with standard vision tests [56]. They also stress that successful translation will require rigorous off-target profiling, careful timing relative to disease progression, and deep-phenotyping pipelines to stratify candidates for personalized intervention [56]. Preclinical evidence supports these findings by showing how CRISPR/Cas9 disruption of the BBS modifier gene Ccdc28b in mice prevented retinal degeneration and obesity but unexpectedly produced autism-like behaviors, emphasizing the complexity of gene–gene interactions in ciliopathies and the value of genome editing for uncovering subtle phenotypic effects [66].

BBS-specific CRISPR therapies remain in the preclinical stage of research. On the other hand, patients with Leber congenital amaurosis due to the CEP290 mutation (LCA10) have been well studied in the clinical trial EDIT-101, where the first in vivo CRISPR therapy has been successfully conducted [67]. This clinical trial is extremely important because it demonstrated a favorable safety profile and visual improvement in early assessments, validating CRISPR as an alternative for subretinal delivery in humans. Sundaresan and co-workers further emphasized how the eye's unique anatomy, accessibility, and immune privilege work as ideal conditions for safe and effective gene editing [68]. They reviewed

CRISPR applications for ocular diseases, noting its precision and potential durability when correcting causal mutations in photoreceptors or retinal pigment epithelial cells. Altay and co-workers highlight that CRISPR derivatives such as base and prime editors provide greater specificity and fewer off-target effects for retinal gene editing in BBS [69]. The review by Jo and co-workers reinforces this by showing in-animal models of retinitis pigmentosa and Leber congenital amaurosis that these editors can repair mutations without double-strand breaks, improve vision, and be delivered successfully via split-AAV or non-viral vectors, a possible approach that could likewise correct many single mutations in BBS genes [69,70].

Currently, no clinical trials of gene editing have been initiated for BBS or other retinal ciliopathies; all available data are derived from preclinical animal models or in vitro systems, with the notable exception of EDIT-101 that serves as an important precedent for in vivo retinal gene editing in humans [67]. While gene editing offers considerable potential for mutation-specific correction, all current CRISPR-based therapies for BBS remain in the preclinical stage, and rigorous off-target profiling, as well as long-term safety assessments, will be essential prerequisites before initiating human trials.

5.3. Pharmacologic Approach—Nonsense Suppression Therapy

One targeted approach currently under investigation is nonsense suppression therapy, also known as readthrough therapy. This strategy aims to treat genetic mutations that introduce premature stop codons by enabling the cellular translation machinery to bypass the stop signal and produce a full-length, functional protein [71]. Nonsense mutations account for approximately 11% of disease-causing variants in BBS, leading to truncated and non-functional ciliary proteins that contribute to retinal degeneration [72,73]. Several pharmacologic agents have demonstrated readthrough activity in cell and animal models of other genetic disorders, including cystic fibrosis and Duchenne's muscular dystrophy [74–76]. Additionally, newer translational readthrough-inducing drugs (TRIDs) have been explored in choroideremia, Usher syndrome, and retinitis pigmentosa type 2 [77–79]. In the context of BBS, Eintracht and co-workers conducted the first study using TRIDs in patients with BBS-derived cells [73]. Fibroblasts from a patient with *BBS2* nonsense mutations treated with ataluren or amlexanox showed restored production of the full-length BBS2 protein to approximately 35–40% of normal levels [73]. These drugs were also able to rescue ciliogenesis and cellular function in fibroblasts, suggesting that nonsense suppression therapy may hold promise for restoring protein expression and ciliary activity in cells of patients with BBS [73].

5.4. Antioxidant and Neuroprotective Therapies

The retinal degeneration observed in patients with BBS has been linked to increased oxidative stress, which is hypothesized to contribute to disease progression [80]. Elevated levels of mitochondrial fluorescent flavoproteins have been detected in the retinas of patients with BBS. It serves as a biomarker of oxidative stress [80]. Antioxidant therapies have therefore been investigated as a potential strategy to mitigate photoreceptor degeneration. In a *BBS10* knock-out mouse model, oral administration of N-acetylcysteine (NAC) preserved retinal structure and function [81]. Treated mice showed significantly thicker outer nuclear layers, improved electroretinogram (ERG) b-wave amplitudes, enhanced photoreceptor synaptic connectivity, and reduced oxidative stress markers compared to untreated controls [81].

Neuroprotective therapies are interventions designed to preserve neuronal integrity, prevent apoptosis, and maintain the functional capacity of cells under disease-related stress. These therapies are particularly important for patients with the syndrome because they can potentially mitigate photoreceptor death caused by ciliary dysfunction, thereby preserving vision [8,82]. One class of neuroprotective agents includes chemical chaperones, which reduce endoplasmic reticulum (ER) stress and protein misfolding, two contributors to photoreceptor apoptosis [83]. In *BBS1^M390R/M390R^* knock-in mice, the bile acid derivative tauroursodeoxycholic acid (TUDCA) preserved photoreceptor OS and maintained ERG responses compared to untreated controls [83]. TUDCA-treated mice also avoided obesity, another phenotype of the model, highlighting both retinal and systemic benefits [83]. Notably, both the NAC and TUDCA findings are derived from murine models of BBS, and although they demonstrate structural and functional preservation in photoreceptors, no human clinical trials have been conducted to date, underscoring the need for further translational validation before clinical application.

Another emerging neuroprotective treatment for patients with BBS involves the DNA damage response (DDR). Barabino and co-workers found that retinal progenitor cells and cone photoreceptors derived from a patient with the BBS10 mutation exhibited persistent DDR activation through the ATM/ATR-Chk2 checkpoint pathway [84]. This stress response contributed to early photoreceptor degeneration. Treatment with a Chk2 kinase inhibitor significantly improved tissue lamination, cone survival, and OS maturation in patient-derived retinal organoids, supporting the role of DDR modulation as a therapeutic avenue in BBS-associated retinal dystrophy [84]. Despite encouraging preclinical results, no human trials have yet been initiated for these pharmacologic or neuroprotective therapies in BBS, and translation into clinical practice will require thorough evaluation of efficacy, optimal dosing, safety, and long-term effects in prospective studies.

6. Current Standard Ophthalmologic Work-Up and Management in Patients with BBS

6.1. Ophthalmologic Work-Up of Patients with BBS

Patients with BBS require age-specific and longitudinal ophthalmologic assessments due to the progressive nature of their retinal and ocular manifestations. In infants and young children, initial evaluation should include screening for strabismus and nystagmus, along with an assessment of visual acuity using age-appropriate methods such as preferential looking or Teller acuity cards in preverbal children, and Snellen charts in older children [17,40]. In adults, visual acuity is evaluated using Snellen charts, and formal cataract assessment with slit-lamp examination is recommended [17]. Visual fields are assessed with Goldmann kinetic perimetry, tailored to the patient's age and degree of remaining vision [40]. Cycloplegic refraction, conducted according to age-specific guidelines, is essential for determining best corrected visual acuity (BCVA) [40]. Given the high prevalence of refractive errors in patients with BBS, regular follow-up refractions are advised, and full optical correction should be prescribed unless visual function is no longer detectable [40]. Fundus photography is useful for evaluating retinal changes and optic nerve appearance and is often feasible even in younger patients [40]. Advanced imaging modalities such as optical coherence tomography (OCT) can detect outer retinal thinning and photoreceptor loss in patients who can maintain fixation, while fundus autofluorescence (FAF) helps assess retinal pigment epithelium damage, often showing a peri-macular hyper autofluorescence ring as a marker of active degeneration [40]. Follow-up care in these patients is life-long and multidisciplinary. Expert consensus recommends that children and adults with progressive disease undergo annual ophthalmologic evaluations, including visual acuity, cycloplegic refraction, OCT, and where possible, Goldmann visual field testing and FAF. In contrast, children and adults with stable visual findings may undergo follow-up every two years, although routine monitoring in adults for cataract progression, low-vision needs, and psychosocial adjustment should remain integral to care [17,40].

6.2. Management of Retinal Degeneration in BBS

As there is currently no available therapy that can stop the retinal degeneration in patients with BBS, clinical management is therefore supportive. Current treatment focuses on low-vision rehabilitation and adaptive strategies [40]. Patients are provided with low-vision aids (magnifiers and electronic devices) to maximize use of residual vision [40]. Orientation and mobility training are introduced early, and Braille instruction and other adaptive living skills are encouraged early at diagnosis to prepare for eventual visual deterioration [40]. Assistive tools such as white canes, guide dogs, large-print materials, and voice-recognition software can further help maintain independence as vision loss progresses [40].

Early referral to multidisciplinary support services is essential, particularly for pediatric patients, to facilitate visual development, educational access, and psychosocial adjustment [17,40]. Integration of low-vision specialists, occupational therapists, special education professionals, and mental health providers can substantially improve quality of life and functional outcomes [17,40]. Ongoing collaboration between ophthalmology and other allied fields is critical in managing progressive visual decline and in tailoring care to each patient's evolving needs.

6.3. Management of Other Ophthalmologic Manifestations in BBS

Effective attention and care of other ocular issues in patients with BBS (strabismus, nystagmus, refractive errors, and cataracts) requires a supportive, interdisciplinary approach. While there is no specific cure for the sensory nystagmus in BBS, standard treatments for strabismus are applied—this includes correcting any refractive error with glasses and performing strabismus surgery when needed to improve ocular alignment and binocular function [40]. Refractive errors are extremely common and are managed with appropriate spectacles or contact lenses to optimize visual acuity [40]. Tinted eyeglasses with photoselective filters may be prescribed to reduce photophobia in these patients [40]. Additionally, vision therapy or the use of low-vision aids may be considered to help manage nystagmus-related visual instability and improve functional vision. When cataracts become visually significant, lens extraction with intraocular lens implantation is performed to improve the remaining vision [40]. However, in patients with BBS, visual outcomes following cataract surgery are highly variable and depend largely on the degree of pre-existing retinal degeneration. While some patients may experience improved contrast sensitivity or modest gains in visual acuity, others may not benefit substantially due to advanced photoreceptor loss [17,49]. Moreover, postoperative counseling should emphasize that while cataract removal may improve clarity, it does not alter the course of retinal disease, and visual expectations should be tailored accordingly.

7. Discussion

This review highlights that retinal degeneration is among the most consistent and earliest clinical features in patients with BBS. Notably, the pattern of degeneration often involves early macular involvement, which distinguishes BBS from other inherited retinal disorders such as nonsyndromic retinitis pigmentosa. As a result, central vision tends to be compromised at an early stage, affecting functional vision and contributing to more severe visual impairment in these patients. This hallmark macular involvement supports the rationale for routine macular imaging in pediatric patients and underscores the need for early initiation of low-vision rehabilitation to optimize developmental and educational outcomes.

Another important aspect of BBS is the genotype–phenotype correlations. Studies have shown that mutations in BBS10 are typically associated with an earlier onset and more rapid progression of visual impairment compared to those with a mutation in BBS1. Therefore, identifying the specific genetic variant is crucial during diagnosis as it can offer valuable prognostic and therapeutic information for the optimal management of these patients. In clinical practice, these correlations support individualized prognostic counseling and guide the frequency and intensity of ophthalmologic follow-up, with BBS10 patients requiring closer monitoring and earlier implementation of low-vision strategies. Still, the literature also emphasizes the marked clinical heterogeneity observed even among patients with the same mutation, suggesting that non-genetic factors may influence phenotypic expression. Despite this variability, there is general agreement that most patients with BBS present with visual dysfunction in early childhood and reach legal blindness by early adulthood. Because of this severe visual impairment during early life and the fact that visual manifestations often precede the diagnosis of other systemic features, ophthalmologists play a key role in early detection and timely referral for multidisciplinary assessment and genetic evaluation.

Even though much of the current literature focuses on retinal degeneration in patients with BBS, additional ophthalmologic manifestations—such as high refractive errors, strabismus, nystagmus, optic nerve abnormalities, and early cataracts—carry significant clinical implications. These findings can further worsen visual acuity if not identified and managed early. For instance, high astigmatism and early-onset myopia or hyperopia, when left uncorrected, may exacerbate visual decline, making timely refractive evaluation and correction essential. Additionally, features such as sensory strabismus, refractive errors, nystagmus, photophobia, and nyctalopia have been described as some of the earliest clinical signs of BBS. This reinforces that these manifestations are not incidental but rather integral components of the syndrome's ophthalmologic profile, warranting early recognition and management by ophthalmologists. Identifying and addressing these secondary findings early is crucial because early intervention can help preserve some visual function, even when there is ongoing progressive retinal degeneration.

From a therapeutic point of view, this review illustrates how BBS has evolved from a condition with no treatment options to one with several promising proof-of-concept interventions aimed at preserving vision. Gene therapy studies targeting mutations in BBS1, BBS4, and BBS10 have shown encouraging results in animal models, demonstrating improved photoreceptor function and preservation of retinal structures. Preclinical models have shown that subretinal delivery of AAV vectors can restore BBS protein expression and correct mislocalized phototransduction proteins, delaying vision loss. However, these studies also highlight important challenges—such as vector delivery limitations and overexpression toxicity—that emphasize the need for precise control of transgene expression before moving on to human trials. Other key translational barriers include immune responses to AAV capsids, variability in dosing tolerability, and the limited predictive value of animal models for human efficacy and safety. Furthermore, current gene therapy candidates that are mutation-specific, such as AXV-101 for the BBS1 M390R variant, limit their broad applicability across the genetically diverse BBS population.

Gene-editing therapies like CRISPR-Cas9 offer a complementary strategy by targeting specific disease-causing mutations at the molecular level. Although gene editing is still in preclinical stages for BBS and no human trials have yet been initiated, early successes in related retinal disorders and the emergence of high-precision tools like base and prime editors make this therapy a promising one for the near future. Despite all the challenges faced, the recent development of a non-human primate model carrying the mutation in BBS7 represents a critical step in the development of therapeutic approaches in a more clinically relevant system.

Besides gene-based therapies, pharmacologic interventions—including nonsense suppression therapy, antioxidant strategies, and DDR pathway modulation—provide an alternative opportunity for those patients that may not qualify for gene-based therapies. Nonsense suppression therapy can be of particular interest for patients with premature stop codons on the BBS protein because these therapies have shown a way to restore full-length protein synthesis. For example, preclinical studies with therapies like ataluren and amlexanox highlight this therapeutic potential, although clinical translation will require validation of efficacy and durability in vivo. In addition to mutation-targeted approaches, therapies aimed at protecting photoreceptors from secondary damage have been studied. Rather than targeting the genetic defect, antioxidant and neuroprotective strategies work by ameliorating cellular damage that contributes to retinal degeneration caused by oxidative stress, protein misfolding, or DNA instability. Such therapies offer a different treatment pathway that can be of therapeutic use across the genetically diverse mutations causing BBS. By having a different mechanism of action, these pharmacologic interventions could be used as adjunctive treatments to gene-based therapies. This offers a distinct path of visual preservation even when genetic mutations cannot be corrected.

However, the systemic delivery of these agents poses important challenges for targeting the retina. The blood–retinal barrier significantly limits the intraocular availability of systemically administered compounds, potentially reducing therapeutic efficacy. In contrast, intraocular administration—such as intravitreal or subretinal injection—may achieve higher local concentrations but involves procedural risks and does not address systemic BBS manifestations. Nonsense suppression agents like aminoglycosides have shown potential for restoring protein synthesis in preclinical models but carry known risks of retinal and cochlear toxicity when delivered systemically or locally at high doses. Similarly, while antioxidants such as N-acetylcysteine have shown retinal benefits in BBS10−/− mouse models, no clinical trials have confirmed their ocular safety or long-term tolerability in humans. These limitations underscore the need for careful consideration of the delivery route, dosing, and toxicity profiles when advancing systemic or intraocular therapies for BBS-related retinal degeneration.

Despite significant advances, many therapeutic approaches for BBS remain in the experimental or preclinical stages. Emphasizing the importance of supportive ophthalmologic care, such as timely refractive correction, low-vision rehabilitation, and cataract surgery, remains the standard of clinical management. However, the field is rapidly evolving, and ophthalmologists are essential for connecting experimental therapies with clinical care through early diagnosis, patient stratification, and involvement in ongoing therapy trials. Such approaches represent encouraging steps toward preserving vision in this patient population.

8. Conclusions

This review emphasizes the importance of early diagnosis and the need for a comprehensive ophthalmologic evaluation in patients with BBS. One of the most significant symptoms of BBS is the early onset of retinal degeneration, which leads to vision loss and disabilities. Other ophthalmologic complications may further compromise vision if not properly recognized and evaluated in a timely manner. While recent advancements in gene-based therapies and pharmacologic strategies show great potential, it is important to note that no disease-modifying treatments for BBS are currently approved, and supportive care remains the standard of management. By implementing genetic testing alongside personalized ophthalmologic care, we can significantly improve patient morbidity and health outcomes.

Recent advancements in gene-based therapies, gene editing, and pharmacologic approaches may provide various methods for preserving visual health and could become standard care for these patients. The current understanding of the pathophysiology and molecular mechanisms of BBS is still evolving, effective therapeutic options remain limited, and significant challenges persist in translating research into clinical practice. As our knowledge of this syndrome continues to grow, the outlook for patients with BBS becomes increasingly hopeful, bringing us closer to effective and potentially transformative treatments.

9. Future Directions

Future directions for BBS research should prioritize the translation of current preclinical studies into safe and effective treatment options for patients with BBS. Gene augmentation shows promise; however, it requires safe and effective delivery methods to minimize toxicity. Major challenges include AAV vector size limitations, achieving efficient transduction of photoreceptors, and minimizing immune responses and off-target effects. The same applies to gene editing—we need to further understand how to deliver it in vivo and assess its long-term effects. Pharmacologic approaches still need to be adequately validated to understand their true potential as most studies remain in the preclinical stages. Future research should involve more patients and active collaboration with ophthalmologists to report ocular findings. This will help build a more complete picture of the ocular manifestations of BBS and ultimately allow us to better co-manage these patients. Future research should explore alternative therapies, such as cell transplantation and retinal prosthetic devices in patients with BBS.

Author Contributions: Conceptualization, A.R.; methodology, A.R. and E.R.; software, E.R.; validation, N.I.; formal analysis, A.R.; investigation, A.R.; resources, E.R.; data curation, A.R. and E.R.; writing—original draft preparation, A.R.; writing—review and editing, A.R., E.R., and N.I.; visualization, A.R.; supervision, N.I. All authors have read and agreed to the published version of the manuscript.

Funding: This work was supported by the Department of Ophthalmology, University of Puerto Rico, Medical Sciences Campus.

Conflicts of Interest: The authors declare no conflicts of interest.

References

1. Berbari, N.F.; O'Connor, A.K.; Haycraft, C.J.; Yoder, B.K. The primary cilium as a complex signaling center. *Curr. Biol.* **2009**, *19*, R526–R535. [CrossRef] [PubMed]
2. Goetz, S.C.; Anderson, K.V. The primary cilium: A signalling centre during vertebrate development. *Nat. Rev. Genet.* **2010**, *11*, 331–344. [CrossRef] [PubMed]
3. Christensen, S.T.; Pedersen, L.B.; Satir, P.; Veland, I.R. The primary cilium coordinates signaling pathways in cell cycle control and migration during development and tissue repair. *Curr. Top. Dev. Biol.* **2017**, *123*, 51–86.
4. Reiter, J.F.; Leroux, M.R. Genes and molecular pathways underpinning ciliopathies. *Nat. Rev. Mol. Cell Biol.* **2017**, *18*, 533–547. [CrossRef]
5. Waters, A.M.; Beales, P.L. Ciliopathies: An expanding disease spectrum. *Pediatr. Nephrol.* **2011**, *26*, 1039–1056. [CrossRef]
6. Forsythe, E.; Beales, P.L. Bardet–Biedl syndrome. *Eur. J. Human. Genet.* **2013**, *21*, 8–13. [CrossRef]
7. Mitchison, H.M.; Valente, E.M. Motile and non-motile cilia in human pathology: From function to phenotypes. *J. Pathol.* **2017**, *241*, 294–309. [CrossRef]
8. Mockel, A.; Perdomo, Y.; Stutzmann, F.; Letsch, J.; Marion, V.; Dollfus, H. Retinal dystrophy in Bardet–Biedl syndrome and related syndromic ciliopathies. *Prog. Retin. Eye Res.* **2011**, *30*, 258–274. [CrossRef]
9. Hjortshøj, T.D.; Grønskov, K.; Philp, A.R.; Nishimura, D.Y.; Riise, R.; Sheffield, V.C.; Brøndum-Nielsen, K. Bardet–Biedl syndrome in Denmark—Report of 13 novel sequence variations in six genes. *Human. Mutat.* **2009**, *31*, 429–436. [CrossRef]
10. Beales, P.L.; Elcioglu, N.; Woolf, A.S.; Parker, D.; Flinter, F.A. New criteria for improved diagnosis of Bardet–Biedl syndrome: Results of a population survey. *J. Med. Genet.* **1999**, *36*, 437–446. [CrossRef]
11. Birtel, J.; Gliem, M.; Herrmann, P. Genotype–phenotype correlations in Bardet–Biedl syndrome. *Eye* **2022**, *36*, 1234–1242.
12. Esposito, M.; Chakarova, C.; Khanna, H. Phenotypic variability in BBS: Insights from retinal imaging. *Mol. Vis.* **2021**, *27*, 415–425.
13. Moore, A.T.; Racher, H.; Holder, G.E. Ocular features in Bardet–Biedl syndrome: Insights from electrodiagnostics and retinal imaging. *Ophthalmic Genet.* **2022**, *43*, 138–145.

14. Milibari, D.; Nowilaty, S.R.; Ba-Abbad, R. The Clinical and Mutational Spectrum of Bardet-Biedl Syndrome in Saudi Arabia. *Genes* **2024**, *15*, 762. [CrossRef]
15. Braun, D.A.; Hildebrandt, F. Ciliopathies. *Cold Spring Harb. Perspect. Biol.* **2022**, *14*, a039214. [CrossRef]
16. Delvallée, C.; Dollfus, H. Retinal ciliopathies: Clinical spectrum and molecular mechanisms. *Int. J. Mol. Sci.* **2023**, *24*, 3981.
17. Forsyth, R.; Gunay-Aygun, M. *Bardet-Biedl Syndrome Overview*; GeneReviews® [Internet]: Seattle, WA, USA, 2023.
18. Álvarez-Satta, M.; Castro-Sánchez, S.; Valverde, D. Bardet–Biedl syndrome as a chaperonopathy: Dissecting the major role of chaperonin-like BBS proteins (BBS6, BBS10 and BBS12). *J. Cell. Mol. Med.* **2017**, *21*, 278–287. [CrossRef]
19. Baker, K.; Beales, P.L. Making sense of cilia in disease: The human ciliopathies. *Am. J. Med. Genet. Part C Semin. Med. Genet.* **2009**, *151C*, 281–295. [CrossRef]
20. Zhou, C.; Deretic, D. The role of the BBSome in photoreceptor membrane protein trafficking and retinal degeneration. *Front. Cell Dev. Biol.* **2022**, *10*, 833334.
21. Hsu, Y.; Chuang, J.Z.; Sung, C.H. Photoreceptor cilia and retinal ciliopathies. *Nat. Rev. Neurosci.* **2022**, *23*, 440–456.
22. Masek, M.; Etard, C.; Hofmann, C.; Hülsmeier, A.J.; Zang, J.; Takamiya, M.; Gesemann, M.; Neuhauss, S.C.F.; Hornemann, T.; Strähle, U.; et al. Loss of the Bardet-Biedl protein Bbs1 alters photoreceptor outer segment protein and lipid composition. *Nat. Commun.* **2022**, *13*, 1282. [CrossRef]
23. Bales, K.L.; Bentley, M.R.; Croyle, M.J.; Kesterson, R.A.; Yoder, B.K.; Gross, A.K. BBSome Component BBS5 Is Required for Cone Photoreceptor Protein Trafficking and Outer Segment Maintenance. *Invest. Ophthalmol. Vis. Sci.* **2020**, *61*, 17. [CrossRef]
24. Datta, P.; Allamargot, C.; Hudson, J.S.; Andersen, E.K.; Bhattarai, S.; Drack, A.V.; Sheffield, V.C.; Seo, S. Accumulation of non-outer segment proteins in the outer segment underlies photoreceptor degeneration in Bardet-Biedl syndrome. *Proc. Natl. Acad. Sci. USA* **2015**, *112*, E4400–E4409. [CrossRef]
25. Grudzinska Pechhacker, A.; Mayer, A.K.; Strom, T.M.; Weber, B.H.F. Genotype–phenotype correlations in Bardet–Biedl syndrome: Insights from patient-derived iPSC models. *Mol. Genet. Genom. Med.* **2021**, *9*, e1783.
26. Mayer, A.K.; Rohrschneider, K.; Strom, T.M.; Kohl, S. Early-onset retinal degeneration in Bbs10-deficient mice: Implications for treatment in Bardet–Biedl syndrome. *Human. Mol. Genet.* **2022**, *31*, 1050–1063.
27. Denniston, A.K.; Murray, P.I. *Oxford Handbook of Ophthalmology*; Oxford University Press: Oxford, UK, 2014.
28. Forsythe, R.; Racher, H.; Gunay-Aygun, M. Ocular manifestations in Bardet–Biedl syndrome: Genotype–phenotype correlations and disease mechanisms. *Ophthalmic Genet.* **2022**, *43*, 123–134.
29. Berezovsky, A.; Rocha, D.M.; Sacai, P.Y.; Watanabe, S.S.; Cavascan, N.N.; Salomão, S.R. Visual acuity and retinal function in patients with Bardet-Biedl syndrome. *Clinics* **2012**, *67*, 145–149. [CrossRef]
30. Nasser, F.; El-Shanti, H.; Green, J. Electroretinography in syndromic retinal degeneration. *Clin. Ophthalmol.* **2022**, *16*, 3173–3180.
31. Abi Karam, M.; Kovach, J.L. Bull's-eye maculopathy in Bardet–Biedl syndrome: A case report. *JAMA Ophthalmol. Case Rep.* **2023**, *11*, e235894.
32. Milibari, D. Retinal features in Bardet–Biedl syndrome: A retrospective study. *Saudi J. Ophthalmol.* **2022**, *36*, 281–288.
33. Riise, R.; Greenstein, V.C.; Acton, R. Electrophysiologic studies in Bardet–Biedl syndrome. *Br. J. Ophthalmol.* **1996**, *80*, 506–510.
34. Castro-Sánchez, S.; Álvarez-Satta, M.; Valverde, D. Modifier genes and clinical variability in Bardet–Biedl syndrome. *Orphanet J. Rare Dis.* **2015**, *10*, 128.
35. Badano, J.L.; Kim, J.C.; Hoskins, B.E.; Lewis, R.A.; Ansley, S.J.; Cutler, D.J.; Castellan, C.; Beales, P.L.; Leroux, M.R.; Katsanis, N. Heterozygous mutations in BBS1, BBS2 and BBS6 have a potential epistatic effect on Bardet–Biedl patients with two mutations at a second BBS locus. *Human. Mol. Genet.* **2003**, *12*, 1651–1659. [CrossRef]
36. Song, T.; Zhao, Y.; Yu, H. Primary cilium in corneal development and disease. *Exp. Eye Res.* **2023**, *225*, 109330.
37. Yavuz Saricay, Y.; Aydin, R.; Sahin, A. Corneal astigmatism and refractive profile in patients with Bardet–Biedl syndrome. *J. Pediatr. Ophthalmol. Strabismus* **2024**, *61*, 78–84.
38. Monika, K.; Fischer, M.D.; Schmid, M. Genotype–phenotype correlations in refractive error profiles among Bardet–Biedl syndrome patients. *Ophthalmic Genet.* **2023**, *44*, 221–229.
39. Héon, E.; Kim, G.; Qin, N.; Tavares, E.; Vincent, A. Genetic analysis of Bardet–Biedl syndrome genes in a cohort of patients reveals genotype–phenotype correlations. *Am. J. Human. Genet.* **2005**, *76*, 381–390.
40. Dollfus, H.; Chassaing, N.; Faivre, L. Bardet-Biedl syndrome improved diagnosis criteria and management: Inter European Reference Networks consensus statement and recommendations. *Eur. J. Human. Genet.* **2024**, *32*, 1347–1360. [CrossRef]
41. Berezovsky, A.; Shelef, I.; Shalev, S. Ophthalmic manifestations of Bardet–Biedl syndrome in a cohort of Israeli patients. *Isr. Med. Assoc. J.* **2012**, *14*, 568–572.
42. Spaggiari, E.; Cioni, G.; Fazzi, E. Pediatric ophthalmologic findings in Bardet–Biedl syndrome: A multicenter retrospective study. *BMC Ophthalmol.* **2021**, *21*, 189.
43. Khan, S.A.; Muhammad, N.; Khan, M.A.; Kamal, A.; Rehman, Z.U.; Khan, S. Genetics of human Bardet-Biedl syndrome, an updates. *Clin. Genet.* **2016**, *90*, 3–15. [CrossRef]

44. Nasser, F.; Kohl, S.; Kurtenbach, A.; Kempf, M.; Biskup, S.; Zuleger, T.; Haack, T.B.; Weisschuh, N.; Stingl, K.; Zrenner, E. Ophthalmic and Genetic Features of Bardet Biedl Syndrome in a German Cohort. *Genes* **2022**, *13*, 1218. [CrossRef]
45. Gao, S.; Zhang, Q.; Ding, Y.; Wang, L.; Li, Z.; Hu, F.; Yao, R.E.; Yu, T.; Chang, G.; Wang, X. Molecular and phenotypic characteristics of Bardet-Biedl syndrome in Chinese patients. *Orphanet J. Rare Dis.* **2024**, *19*, 149. [CrossRef]
46. Grudzinska Pechhacker, M.K.; Jacobson, S.G.; Drack, A.V.; Scipio, M.D.; Strubbe, I.; Pfeifer, W.; Duncan, J.L.; Dollfus, H.; Goetz, N.; Muller, J.; et al. Comparative Natural History of Visual Function From Patients with Biallelic Variants in BBS1 and BBS10. *Investig. Ophthalmol. Vis. Sci.* **2021**, *62*, 26. [CrossRef]
47. Dollfus, H.; Chassaing, N.; Faivre, L. Bardet–Biedl syndrome: Developmental eye defects and clinical heterogeneity. *Dev. Ophthalmol.* **2020**, *57*, 58–72.
48. Sridhar, S.; Palanivel, S.; Senthilkumar, J.; Kavitha, K.; Geethaanjali, V.; Vasanthiy, N.; Dharmaraj, C. Clinical Presentation and Co-Morbidities in Bardet-Biedel Syndrome: Case Series from a Single Centre. *Indian J. Endocrinol. Metab.* **2025**, *29*, 89–94. [CrossRef]
49. Iannaccone, A.; De Propris, G.; Roncati, S.; Rispoli, E.; Del Porto, G.; Pannarale, M.R. The ocular phenotype of the Bardet-Biedl syndrome. Comparison to non-syndromic retinitis pigmentosa. *Ophthalmic Genet.* **1997**, *18*, 13–26. [CrossRef]
50. Belkadi, A.; Thareja, G.; Khan, A.; Stephan, N.; Zaghlool, S.; Halama, A.; Ahmed, A.A.; Mohamoud, Y.A.; Malek, J.; Suhre, K.; et al. Retinal nerve fibre layer thinning and corneal nerve loss in patients with Bardet-Biedl syndrome. *BMC Med. Genom.* **2023**, *16*, 301. [CrossRef]
51. Chattannavar, G.; Ger, M.; Balasubramanian, J.; Mandal, S.; Jalali, S.; Takkar, B.; Pisuchpen, P.; de Guimaraes, T.A.C.; Capasso, J.E.; Kumar Padhy, S.; et al. Bardet-Biedl syndrome with chorioretinal coloboma: A case series and review of literature. *Ophthalmic Genet.* **2024**, *45*, 616–622. [CrossRef]
52. Barwar, G.; Parchand, S.M.; Gangwe, A.B.; Agrawal, D. A rare combination: Bardet–Biedl syndrome with atypical retinitis pigmentosa and optic disc drusen. *Indian J. Ophthalmol. -Case Rep.* **2023**, *3*, 396–398. [CrossRef]
53. American Society of Gene and Cell Therapy. Gene Therapy Basics. Available online: https://patienteducation.asgct.org/gene-therapy-101/gene-therapy-basics (accessed on 20 May 2025).
54. Simons, D.L.; Boye, S.L.; Hauswirth, W.W.; Wu, S.M. Gene therapy prevents photoreceptor death and preserves retinal function in a Bardet-Biedl syndrome mouse model. *Proc. Natl. Acad. Sci. USA* **2011**, *108*, 6276–6281. [CrossRef]
55. Seo, S.; Mullins, R.F.; Dumitrescu, A.V.; Bhattarai, S.; Gratie, D.; Wang, K.; Stone, E.M.; Sheffield, V.; Drack, A.V. Subretinal gene therapy of mice with Bardet-Biedl syndrome type 1. *Invest. Ophthalmol. Vis. Sci.* **2013**, *54*, 6118–6132. [CrossRef] [PubMed]
56. Kenny, J.; Forsythe, E.; Beales, P.; Bacchelli, C. Toward personalized medicine in Bardet-Biedl syndrome. *Pers. Med.* **2017**, *14*, 447–456. [CrossRef]
57. Hsu, Y.; Bhattarai, S.; Thompson, J.M.; Mahoney, A.; Thomas, J.; Mayer, S.K.; Datta, P.; Garrison, J.; Searby, C.C.; Vandenberghe, L.H.; et al. Subretinal gene therapy delays vision loss in a Bardet-Biedl Syndrome type 10 mouse model. *Mol. Ther. Nucleic Acids* **2023**, *31*, 164–181. [CrossRef]
58. Peterson, S.M.; McGill, T.J.; Puthussery, T.; Stoddard, J.; Renner, L.; Lewis, A.D.; Colgin, L.M.A.; Gayet, J.; Wang, X.; Prongay, K.; et al. Bardet-Biedl Syndrome in rhesus macaques: A nonhuman primate model of retinitis pigmentosa. *Exp. Eye Res.* **2019**, *189*, 107825. [CrossRef]
59. Foundation, B.B.S. Clinical Practice. Available online: https://www.bardetbiedl.org/clinical-practice (accessed on 16 May 2025).
60. Axovia Therapeutics. AXV-101: A Gene Therapy for BBS1-Related Retinal Degeneration. 2024. Available online: https://www.axoviatherapeutics.com/pipeline/axv-101 (accessed on 12 May 2025).
61. Molinari, E.; Sayer, J.A. Gene and epigenetic editing in the treatment of primary ciliopathies. *Prog. Mol. Biol. Transl. Sci.* **2021**, *182*, 353–401.
62. Jinek, M.; Chylinski, K.; Fonfara, I.; Hauer, M.; Doudna, J.A.; Charpentier, E. A Programmable Dual-RNA–Guided DNA Endonuclease in Adaptive Bacterial Immunity. *Science* **2012**, *337*, 816–821. [CrossRef]
63. Doudna, J.A.; Charpentier, E. The new frontier of genome engineering with CRISPR-Cas9. *Science* **2014**, *346*, 1258096. [CrossRef]
64. Sternberg, S.H.; Doudna, J.A. Expanding the Biologist's Toolkit with CRISPR-Cas9. *Mol. Cell* **2015**, *58*, 568–574. [CrossRef]
65. Ahmad, I. CRISPR/Cas9—A Promising Therapeutic Tool to Cure Blindness: Current Scenario and Future Prospects. *Int. J. Mol. Sci.* **2022**, *23*, 11482. [CrossRef] [PubMed]
66. Fabregat, M.; Niño-Rivero, S.; Pose, S.; Cárdenas-Rodríguez, M.; Bresque, M.; Hernández, K.; Prieto-Echagüe, V.; Schlapp, G.; Crispo, M.; Lagos, P.; et al. Generation and characterization of Ccdc28b mutant mice links the Bardet-Biedl associated gene with mild social behavioral phenotypes. *PLoS Genet.* **2022**, *18*, e1009896. [CrossRef] [PubMed]
67. Suh, S.; Choi, E.H.; Raguram, A.; Liu, D.R.; Palczewski, K. Precision genome editing in the eye. *Proc. Natl. Acad. Sci. USA* **2022**, *119*, e2210104119. [CrossRef] [PubMed]
68. Sundaresan, Y.; Yacoub, S.; Kodati, B.; Amankwa, C.E.; Raola, A.; Zode, G. Therapeutic applications of CRISPR/Cas9 gene editing technology for the treatment of ocular diseases. *FEBS J.* **2023**, *290*, 5248–5269. [CrossRef]

69. Altay, H.Y.; Ozdemir, F.; Afghah, F.; Kilinc, Z.; Ahmadian, M.; Tschopp, M.; Agca, C. Gene regulatory and gene editing tools and their applications for retinal diseases and neuroprotection: From proof-of-concept to clinical trial. *Front. Neurosci.* **2022**, *16*, 924917. [CrossRef]
70. Jo, D.H.; Bae, S.; Kim, H.H.; Kim, J.S.; Kim, J.H. In vivo application of base and prime editing to treat inherited retinal diseases. *Prog. Retin. Eye Res.* **2023**, *94*, 101132. [CrossRef]
71. Richardson, R.; Smart, M.; Tracey-White, D.; Webster, A.R.; Moosajee, M. Mechanism and evidence of nonsense suppression therapy for genetic eye disorders. *Exp. Eye Res.* **2017**, *155*, 24–37. [CrossRef] [PubMed]
72. Forsythe, E.; Kenny, J.; Bacchelli, C.; Beales, P.L. Managing Bardet-Biedl Syndrome-Now and in the Future. *Front. Pediatr.* **2018**, *6*, 23. [CrossRef]
73. Eintracht, J.; Forsythe, E.; May-Simera, H.; Moosajee, M. Translational readthrough of ciliopathy genes BBS2 and ALMS1 restores protein, ciliogenesis and function in patient fibroblasts. *EBioMedicine* **2021**, *70*, 103515. [CrossRef]
74. Mutyam, V.; Du, M.; Xue, X.; Keeling, K.M.; White, E.L.; Bostwick, J.R.; Rasmussen, L.; Liu, B.; Mazur, M.; Hong, J.S.; et al. Discovery of Clinically Approved Agents That Promote Suppression of Cystic Fibrosis Transmembrane Conductance Regulator Nonsense Mutations. *Am. J. Respir. Crit. Care Med.* **2016**, *194*, 1092–1103. [CrossRef]
75. Xue, X.; Mutyam, V.; Thakerar, A.; Mobley, J.; Bridges, R.J.; Rowe, S.M.; Keeling, K.M.; Bedwell, D.M. Identification of the amino acids inserted during suppression of CFTR nonsense mutations and determination of their functional consequences. *Hum. Mol. Genet.* **2017**, *26*, 3116–3129. [CrossRef]
76. Finkel, R.S.; Flanigan, K.M.; Wong, B.; Bönnemann, C.; Sampson, J.; Sweeney, H.L.; Reha, A.; Northcutt, V.J.; Elfring, G.; Barth, J.; et al. Phase 2a Study of Ataluren-Mediated Dystrophin Production in Patients with Nonsense Mutation Duchenne Muscular Dystrophy. *PLoS ONE* **2013**, *8*, e81302. [CrossRef]
77. Tracey-White, D.; De Luca, V.; Futter, C.; Moore, A.T.; Webster, A.; Seabra, M.C.; Hamel, C.P.; Kalatzis, V.; Moosajee, M. Translational bypass therapy using ataluren to treat nonsense-mediated choroideremia. *Investig. Ophthalmol. Vis. Sci.* **2014**, *55*, 3302.
78. Samanta, A.; Stingl, K.; Kohl, S.; Ries, J.; Linnert, J.; Nagel-Wolfrum, K. Ataluren for the Treatment of Usher Syndrome 2A Caused by Nonsense Mutations. *Int. J. Mol. Sci.* **2019**, *20*, 6274. [CrossRef] [PubMed]
79. Schwarz, N.; Carr, A.J.; Lane, A.; Moeller, F.; Chen, L.L.; Aguilà, M.; Nommiste, B.; Muthiah, M.N.; Kanuga, N.; Wolfrum, U.; et al. Translational read-through of the RP2 Arg120stop mutation in patient iPSC-derived retinal pigment epithelium cells. *Hum. Mol. Genet.* **2015**, *24*, 972–986. [CrossRef]
80. Russell, M.W.; Muste, J.C.; Seth, K.; Kumar, M.; Rich, C.A.; Singh, R.P.; Traboulsi, E.I. Functional imaging of mitochondria in genetically confirmed retinal dystrophies using flavoprotein fluorescence. *Ophthalmic Genet.* **2022**, *43*, 834–840. [CrossRef] [PubMed]
81. Rankin, T.; Mayer, S.; Laird, J.; Lobeck, B.; Kalmanek, E.; Drack, A. N-Acetylcysteine Ameliorates Loss of the Electroretinogram b-wave in a Bardet-Biedl Syndrome Type 10 Mouse Model. *J. Exp. Neurol.* **2025**, *6*, 49–63. [CrossRef]
82. Ferraguti, G.; Terracina, S.; Micangeli, G.; Lucarelli, M.; Tarani, L.; Ceccanti, M.; Spaziani, M.; D'Orazi, V.; Petrella, C.; Fiore, M. NGF and BDNF in pediatrics syndromes. *Neurosci. Biobehav. Rev.* **2023**, *145*, 105015. [CrossRef]
83. Drack, A.V.; Dumitrescu, A.V.; Bhattarai, S.; Gratie, D.; Stone, E.M.; Mullins, R.; Sheffield, V.C. TUDCA slows retinal degeneration in two different mouse models of retinitis pigmentosa and prevents obesity in Bardet-Biedl syndrome type 1 mice. *Investig. Ophthalmol. Vis. Sci.* **2012**, *53*, 100–106. [CrossRef]
84. Barabino, A.; Katbe, A.; Hanna, R.; Freedman, B.S.; Bernier, G. Pharmaceutical inhibition of the Chk2 kinase mitigates cone photoreceptor degeneration in an iPSC model of Bardet-Biedl syndrome. *iScience* **2025**, *28*, 112130. [CrossRef]

medicina

MDPI

Review

Combined Cataract and Vitrectomy Surgery in Pediatric Patients

Armando J. Ruiz-Justiz [1,*], Vanessa Cruz-Villegas [1], Stephen G. Schwartz [2], Victor M. Villegas [1,2,*] and Timothy G. Murray [3,*]

[1] Department of Ophthalmology, University of Puerto Rico School of Medicine, San Juan, PR 00936, USA; vcruz02@msn.com
[2] Department of Ophthalmology, Bascom Palmer Eye Institute, University of Miami Miller School of Medicine, Miami, FL 33136, USA; sschwartz2@med.miami.edu
[3] Miami Ocular Oncology & Retina (MOOR), Miami, FL 33143, USA
* Correspondence: armando.ruiz1@upr.edu (A.J.R.-J.); victor.villegas@upr.edu (V.M.V.); tmurray@murraymd.com (T.G.M.)

Abstract: *Purpose:* To review the current literature on the combined use of cataract surgery (or lensectomy) and vitrectomy in pediatric patients, with a focus on clinical indications, surgical techniques, outcomes, and complications across various pediatric ocular pathologies. *Methods:* A narrative review of published studies addressing the use of combined lensectomy and vitrectomy (LV) in pediatric patients was conducted. Conditions discussed include congenital cataracts, ectopia lentis, retinopathy of prematurity (ROP), retinal detachment (RD), and persistent fetal vasculature (PFV). Key surgical considerations, visual and anatomical outcomes, and postoperative complications were examined. *Results:* The literature search yielded a total of 160 articles, of which 43 met the inclusion criteria and were included in this review. Although lens-sparing vitrectomy (LSV) is preferred in many pediatric cases to preserve accommodation and reduce complications, combined LV is often necessary in advanced or complex diseases. Studies have shown that combined LV can achieve favorable anatomical outcomes, but functional visual recovery remains variable and is affected by factors such as patient age, baseline ocular anatomy, and disease severity. Postoperative complications such as glaucoma, visual axis opacification (VAO), and intraocular lens (IOL) dislocation are more frequent with combined procedures and require long-term follow-up and rehabilitation. *Conclusions:* Combined cataract surgery (or lensectomy) and vitrectomy may represent a valuable strategy in the management of complex pediatric ocular conditions, particularly when individualized to the clinical context. Tailored surgical approaches are essential to optimize anatomic and functional outcomes. Further prospective studies and harmonized multicenter registries are needed to develop evidence-based principles that can guide individualized surgical decision-making in this unique patient population.

Keywords: lensectomy-vitrectomy; congenital cataracts; ectopia lentis; retinopathy of prematurity; retinal detachment; persistent fetal vasculature

1. Introduction

The use of combined cataract surgery (or lensectomy) and vitrectomy in pediatric patients is not well-documented in the current medical literature. Although numerous studies have evaluated pars plana vitrectomy (PPV) techniques and outcomes in children, few have specifically addressed the combined approach of cataract extraction or lensectomy with vitrectomy in this population.

Cataract surgery has advanced considerably over the past few decades, particularly with the widespread adoption of phacoemulsification in adult patients. However, pediatric cataract surgery poses unique anatomical and physiological challenges that require different surgical strategies [1]. Unlike adults, phacoemulsification is not the preferred technique for pediatric patients due to the softness of the crystalline lens and the increased risk of complications [1]. In this group, the lens can typically be removed using manual irrigation and aspiration or vitrector-assisted lensectomy, thereby avoiding the need for ultrasonic energy [2]. Moreover, pediatric eyes present with a smaller anterior segment, increased zonular laxity, and a more fragile lens capsule, all of which increase surgical complexity [2]. Additional intraoperative considerations such as primary posterior capsulectomy and anterior vitrectomy are often necessary to reduce the high risk of posterior capsule opacification (PCO) [3].

In complex pediatric ocular conditions, combining cataract extraction or lensectomy (either with or without intraocular lens (IOL) implantation) with vitrectomy is commonly employed, as it may offer significant clinical advantages (Figure 1) [4]. Reported benefits include enhanced visualization of the posterior segment, reduced postoperative vitreous traction, lower rates of macular edema, and the ability to consolidate procedures, thereby decreasing the need for multiple surgical interventions [4]. However, this combined approach carries its own risks, including posterior capsular rupture, zonular dialysis, and posterior dislocation of lens fragments [5].

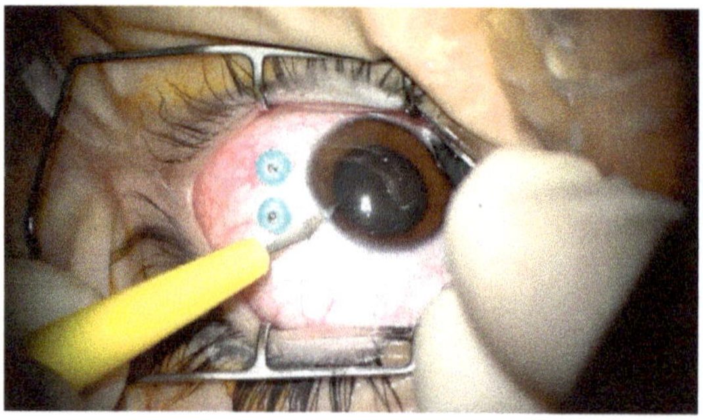

Figure 1. Clear corneal incision in a pediatric patient undergoing combined cataract and vitrectomy surgery.

Several pediatric conditions may necessitate this combined surgical approach, particularly in advanced stages [4]. These include retinopathy of prematurity (ROP), ectopia lentis, retinal detachment (RD), and persistent fetal vasculature (PFV). In such cases, PPV alone or in combination with lensectomy may be required to manage tractional or obstructive pathology [4]. One of the most significant postoperative complications of PPV in pediatric patients is cataract formation, with reported rates as high as 61% [6,7]. This has prompted debate regarding whether a combined lensectomy with IOL implantation and vitrectomy should be preferred over lens-sparing vitrectomy (LSV), particularly in patients at high risk for subsequent cataract development [6,7].

This review aims to summarize the existing literature on the use of combined cataract surgery (or lensectomy) and vitrectomy in pediatric patients, highlighting its indications, advantages, limitations, and clinical outcomes across various pediatric ocular pathologies.

2. Materials and Methods

A literature search was performed using the PubMed (https://pubmed.ncbi.nlm.nih.gov/) and Google Scholar (https://scholar.google.com) databases for articles published up to May 2025. Search terms included combinations of: "pediatric cataract", "lensectomy", "vitrectomy", "pars plana vitrectomy", "lens-sparing vitrectomy", "lensectomy-vitrectomy", "pediatric", "retinopathy of prematurity", "persistent fetal vasculature", "ectopia lentis", and "retinal detachment".

Prospective and retrospective clinical studies, case series, and relevant review articles were considered. Inclusion criteria were studies published in English that addressed combined lensectomy and vitrectomy (combined LV) techniques in pediatric patients for the management of pediatric cataracts, ectopia lentis, ROP, RD, and PFV. Exclusion criteria included studies focused solely on adult patients, animal models, or those not evaluating lensectomy and vitrectomy procedures.

Due to the heterogeneity of study designs, surgical techniques, and outcome measures across the included literature, a systematic review or meta-analysis was not feasible. Instead, findings were qualitatively summarized to identify trends in surgical decision-making, procedural approaches, and clinical outcomes. Comparative tables were constructed to summarize surgical indications for combined LV, IOL strategies, outcomes, and associated complications.

3. Results

The initial literature search yielded a total of 160 articles. After screening titles and abstracts and applying the inclusion and exclusion criteria, 43 articles were deemed relevant and included in this narrative review. Among these, there were 23 retrospective studies, 10 narrative reviews, 4 prospective studies, 3 case reports, 2 systematic reviews, and 1 case series. No randomized controlled trials were identified.

Most studies focused on surgical techniques, visual and anatomical outcomes, and postoperative complications. The majority of clinical studies were conducted at single institutions, with varying sample sizes and follow-up durations.

4. Discussion

4.1. Pediatric Cataract

Pediatric cataracts remain a leading cause of treatable visual impairment in children worldwide [8]. Prevalence estimates range from 0.63 to 13.6 per 10,000 in low-income countries and 0.42 to 2.05 per 10,000 in high-income countries [3]. They are broadly classified into congenital and acquired types [3]. Early surgical intervention is essential to prevent deprivation amblyopia [9]. Despite consensus on the need for early treatment, the optimal timing and surgical approach for pediatric cataract management continue to be debated.

The importance of technique selection and age-specific surgical planning is highlighted in a retrospective study by Li et al. (2023), which evaluated long-term visual outcomes and complications following lensectomy with anterior vitrectomy and primary IOL implantation in children with bilateral congenital cataracts [10]. The study analyzed 148 eyes from 74 patients who underwent surgery via a limbal approach using a 25-gauge micro-incision vitrectomy system. Surgical steps included lensectomy, anterior vitrectomy, and in-the-bag IOL implantation under general anesthesia. The most common postoperative complications requiring reoperation included visual axis opacification (VAO) (5.4%), IOL pupillary capture (2.0%), iris incarceration (0.7%), and glaucoma (0.7%) [10]. Children younger than 2 years demonstrated a higher incidence of VAO and greater postoperative refractive error compared to older age groups [10]. The mean final best-corrected visual acuity (BCVA) was 0.24 $\pm$ 0.32 logMAR, with 22 eyes (14.9%) classified as having low vision (BCVA worse than 0.5 logMAR). These findings suggest that lensectomy with anterior vitrectomy and IOL implantation may be effective and reasonably safe in selected pediatric cases [10].

However, they also underscore the importance of age-specific risk stratification and the need for long-term follow-up, particularly in children under 2 years of age and those with dense cataracts or preexisting comorbidities [10].

VAO is the preferred term over posterior capsule opacification (PCO) in pediatric patients, as visual obscuration can occur despite the creation of a primary posterior capsulorhexis [11]. The underlying pathophysiology of VAO is believed to be either proliferative and/or fibrotic in nature [11]. This includes excessive mitotic activity of residual equatorial lens epithelial cells that migrate into the visual axis, or epithelial-mesenchymal transdifferentiation leading to fibrotic membrane formation. Both mechanisms contribute to visual axis obscuration [11].

Anterior vitrectomy in pediatric cataract surgery plays a pivotal role in reducing postoperative complications, particularly VAO [12]. Kugelberg et al. (2002) demonstrated a statistically significant reduction in reoperation rates due to VAO in children under 7 years old when anterior vitrectomy was performed at the time of cataract surgery [12]. Conversely, a more recent analysis by Yen et al. (2023) did not find age to significantly influence the effectiveness of anterior vitrectomy in preventing VAO, suggesting that the procedure may be beneficial across all pediatric age groups [13].

Postoperative glaucoma is another major complication following cataract surgery in infancy and remains a leading cause of long-term vision loss in this population [14]. Yen et al. (2023) reported that the risk of glaucoma development after anterior vitrectomy and IOL implantation was not significantly associated with patient age [13]. This finding underscores the importance of long-term monitoring for glaucoma in all pediatric patients undergoing cataract surgery, regardless of age or surgical approach [13].

Surgical decision-making in pediatric cataract cases should consider patient age, lens density, and the presence of posterior segment pathology [3,10–15]. Lensectomy with anterior vitrectomy is typically recommended in younger children due to the higher risk of VAO [15].

4.2. Ectopia Lentis

Ectopia lentis in pediatric patients can result from trauma or may occur secondary to systemic conditions such as Marfan syndrome and other connective tissue disorders [16]. Surgical management of ectopia lentis is complex, and the choice of surgical technique is highly case-dependent [16]. Typically, combined LV is performed, with or without IOL implantation, based on patient age, visual potential, and the presence of ocular comorbidities [17]. Various IOL implantation modalities have been developed for these cases, including anterior chamber IOLs, iris-claw or iris-sutured IOLs, sutured scleral-fixated IOLs (SSFIOLs), and posterior chamber IOLs [17].

SSFIOLs have been proposed as an effective means of correcting aphakia in pediatric patients lacking adequate capsular support [18]. In a study by Sen, P. et al. (2018), pediatric patients with congenital or traumatic lens subluxation underwent PPV with lens extraction followed by SSFIOL implantation using a four-point ab externo fixation technique [18]. The IOL implanted was a posterior chamber polymethyl methacrylate (PMMA) lens (Hanita) with a 6.5 mm optic diameter and a 13 mm overall diameter. Postoperative complications included choroidal detachment (2.86%), dispersed vitreous hemorrhage (2.86%), endophthalmitis (0.72%), elevated intraocular pressure (12.54%), diplopia (0.72%), retinal detachment (5.73%), and SSFIOL dislocation (4.6%) [18,19]. Despite these complications, best-corrected visual acuity (BCVA) was maintained or improved in 93.19% of eyes, supporting the effectiveness of this therapeutic approach [18].

Iris-sutures intraocular lenses are another viable surgical option to ensure adequate lens position [20]. Kopel et al. (2008) evaluated 22 eyes from 12 pediatric patients with ectopia lentis who underwent PPV and vitrectomy, with or without implantation of a foldable iris-sutured IOL [20]. All procedures were performed by a single vitreoretinal surgeon between 1998 and 2006. This study demonstrated that iris-fixated IOL implantation yielded visual outcomes comparable to those achieved with optically corrected aphakia, although the risk of IOL dislocation remained a significant concern [20].

In ectopia lentis, the choice of combined LV is primarily driven by the extent of lens instability, degree of capsular support, and age-appropriate IOL considerations [16]. Children with severe subluxation and inadequate zonular support benefit most from combined LV with scleral-fixated or iris-sutured IOLs [16–20].

4.3. *Advanced Retinopathy of Prematurity (ROP)*

ROP remains a leading cause of childhood blindness worldwide, especially in low-birthweight and preterm infants [21]. Early intervention with photocoagulation or intravitreal anti-VEGF therapy can prevent progression in many cases. However, advanced stages (Stage 4A, 4B, and 5 ROP) often require surgical intervention due to tractional retinal detachment (TRD) [21].

Surgical management in advanced cases typically involves vitrectomy or combined LV [22]. The need for lensectomy arises when fibrovascular proliferation extends anteriorly, obscuring the view or limiting access for membrane peeling and adequate traction release, or in cases with significant retrolental fibrosis [22]. When posterior structures can be safely visualized and accessed, LSV is preferred due to better visual and anatomic outcomes [22,23].

Sen et al. (2023) compared LSV and combined LV in a cohort of Stage 4 and 5 ROP eyes, demonstrating that LSV resulted in better visual outcomes and fewer postoperative complications [22]. Additionally, LSV has been associated with a lower incidence of glaucoma and amblyopia [22]. The combined LV group consisted of more complex cases, indicating that the surgical choice often reflects the underlying severity [22]. This is corroborated by data from Chang et al. (2024), who found that anatomic success was highest in Stage 4A (96.3%) and declined in more severe stages, with only 31.3% anatomic success in Stage 5 ROP [24]. Notably, the need for combined LV in Stage 4 eyes was significantly associated with poorer outcomes, suggesting that surgical complexity is a marker of worse prognosis [24].

In particularly severe cases, such as Stage 5C ROP (total retinal detachment along with anterior segment anomalies) with corneal opacification, a staged lensectomy and vitrectomy approach has been proposed [25]. Fei (2022) reported that performing lensectomy first, followed by delayed vitrectomy after corneal clearing, achieved partial retinal reattachment in 63.6% of eyes and restored corneal clarity in the majority, offering a strategic advantage when the posterior segment is initially inaccessible [25]. In this study, regular combined LV was not performed due to the invisible fundus. The average interval between the two procedures was 6.8 ± 4.6 months (2.5–18.5 months).

Modified surgical techniques have also evolved to minimize complications and improve access. Chandra et al. (2019) described a hybrid clear corneal micro-incision lensectomy and vitrectomy approach using 25G instruments in 50 eyes with Stage 5 ROP [26]. Sutureless closure without complications such as hypotony, flat anterior chamber, hyphema, or corneal edema was achieved [26]. This technique has been proposed as a safe and viable surgical alternative for Stage 5 ROP based on limited case series data, decreasing the high risk of iatrogenic breaks due to anterior retinal traction seen in traditional pars plana approaches [26].

Despite surgical advances, long-term complications such as glaucoma remain a concern [27,28]. Chandra (2019) and Nudleman (2017) both reported a higher risk of secondary glaucoma in patients undergoing combined LV, likely due to anterior segment disruption and increased inflammation [27,28]. Even LSV carries a risk, particularly in severe ROP stages [28].

Anatomic reattachment does not always correlate with functional vision [29,30]. Chehaibou et al. (2024) reported macular reattachment in 57.8% of eyes undergoing modified limbal LV, but only 64.1% achieved light perception or better [29]. Similarly, Rishi et al. (2019) presented a long-term follow-up of a patient with excellent anatomical outcome after combined LV who later developed Descemet's membrane detachment 15 years postoperatively, illustrating that late sequelae can still compromise visual rehabilitation [30].

Collectively, the literature emphasizes that the surgical approach should be individualized based on disease stage, anterior segment clarity, and extent of fibrovascular proliferation [21–30]. While LSV remains the preferred option for less advanced disease, combined LV is indispensable in eyes with anterior TRD, retrolental fibrosis, or media opacities [22,23]. However, it must be approached cautiously given its association with poorer visual outcomes and higher postoperative morbidity.

4.4. Retinal Detachment (RD)

Rhegmatogenous retinal detachment (RRD) is a major vision-threatening condition [31]. RRD can result from retinal tears caused by trauma, structural retinal anomalies, pathological myopia, complicated cataract surgery, or posterior vitreous detachment [31]. Although RRD is more common in adults, retinal tears may also occur in younger patients, particularly after trauma or in association with hereditary collagen disorders [32].

Surgical repair of RRD using PPV has an anatomic success rate of approximately 80% [33]. A major complication of PPV in phakic eyes is the progressive development of cataracts, often necessitating cataract surgery, which may be technically more challenging in such cases [31].

LSV is preferred in pediatric patients, especially for cases involving TRD or opaque media [34]. Preserving the natural lens is critical in children to maintain accommodation. Therefore, LSV is often the procedure of choice when possible [31]. A retrospective analysis by Ferrone et al. (1997), which evaluated 85 eyes of 77 pediatric patients, found that 67% of lenses remained clear after LSV, while 15% developed cataracts and 18% required lens removal during subsequent surgery [34]. These findings suggest that LSV is effective in preserving lens clarity in the pediatric population [34].

Despite the advantages of LSV, complex retinal detachment cases in children may require combined LV [35,36]. Mendoza et al. (2025) reported a case of exudative RD in a 15-year-old female with Rubinstein–Taybi Syndrome (RTS) caused by a frameshift mutation in the cyclic AMP response element binding protein (CREBBP), who required combined LV [35]. In addition to classic RTS features (developmental delay, microcephaly, and broad thumbs and toes), the patient exhibited several ophthalmic manifestations, including left temporal retinal exudation, exudative RD, and inferotemporal hemorrhage. Despite initial improvement with multiple sessions of photocoagulation, focal TRD developed, necessitating combined LV. Similarly, Kawaguchi et al. (2025) reported two pediatric cases of RTS who developed TRD, both of whom underwent combined LV with IOL implantation [36]. In one case, retinal reattachment was achieved after three vitrectomies; in the other, reattachment could not be accomplished. Both patients developed poorly controlled glaucoma requiring surgical intervention. These cases highlight the complexity of RD management in RTS patients and suggest that treatment often requires multiple surgical interventions and carries an elevated risk of postoperative refractory glaucoma [35,36].

In pediatric RD, LSV is favored when visualization is adequate [34]. However, combined LV is required in cases with TRD or exudative RD where the lens obstructs access to the vitreous base or posterior pathology [34–36].

4.5. Persistent Fetal Vasculature (PFV)

PFV, previously called persistent hyperplastic primary vitreous (PHPV), is a rare but significant developmental anomaly arising from the failure of regression of the hyaloid vasculature, often leading to a spectrum of anterior and posterior ocular pathologies, including cataract, retrolental fibrovascular membranes, and RD [37]. Surgical intervention is frequently indicated in severe cases, particularly in combined PFV, where both anterior and posterior segments are affected [37]. In such situations, combined LV is often necessary to relieve the traction, clear the visual axis, and prevent further anatomic disruption [37].

Several studies have evaluated the safety and efficacy of combined LV for PFV, highlighting both the technical challenges and the potential for functional rehabilitation [38]. In a case series by Lyu et al. (2020) involving 19 eyes with unilateral combined PFV, patients underwent limbal lensectomy, capsulotomy, anterior vitrectomy, dissection of the retrolental membrane and stalk, and in-the-bag IOL implantation [38]. In this study, 95% of IOLs remained well positioned, and retinal dragging was reversed in all 8 eyes with preoperative peripapillary traction. While 47% of eyes achieved BCVA better than 20/200, poorer outcomes were associated with baseline peripapillary retinopathy, emphasizing the prognostic importance of initial retinal health [38]. These findings underscore the feasibility of combined LV with IOL implantation as an alternative to treat eyes with combined PFV, with long-term refractive monitoring required due to postoperative myopic shift [38].

Similarly, Khurana et al. (2021) reported favorable outcomes in a prospective cohort of 20 children undergoing phacoaspiration with or without IOL implantation, combined with dissection and cauterization of the PFV stalk [39]. Good visual fixation (central, steady, maintained) was achieved in 80% of patients, and no cases of intraoperative bleeding, glaucoma, or retinal detachment occurred [39]. The major complication was VAO, requiring membranectomy in 8 children. Visual outcomes were more guarded in children with microphthalmia, aphakia, or combined PFV, reinforcing the importance of early surgical timing and aggressive amblyopia therapy [39].

Even though anatomic restoration is vital, it does not always lead to visual improvement [37]. Loukovaara et al. (2024) found that despite combined LV surgery to address both anterior and posterior PFV components in pediatric patients with unilateral congenital cataract and PFV, visual outcomes were modest [37]. The best result was a visual acuity of 0.5 (20/40 on the Snellen chart) in one child, while others ranged from finger counting to light perception. Contributing factors included amblyopia, microphthalmia, and macular involvement. Postoperative complications such as secondary cataracts and esotropia were also reported, underscoring the need for careful preoperative evaluation and long-term visual rehabilitation strategies [37].

Age and lens status are pivotal in surgical decision-making [40]. In Huang, H.C. et al. (2023), patients with posterior or combined PFV underwent either LSV or combined LV depending on the extent of anterior segment involvement, such as the presence of cataract or lens opacification that obstructed the visual axis or hindered safe access to the PFV stalk [40]. IOL implantation was avoided in children under 2 years due to higher complication risk and concern for ocular growth interference [40]. Only 26.3% of eyes achieved vision better than counting fingers, while 29% suffered poor outcomes including no light perception. However, a significant benefit of surgery was greater axial elongation in operated eyes, suggesting improved cosmetic outcomes through enhanced ocular growth even when visual rehabilitation was limited [40].

Surgical approach also influences outcomes. In a 20-year retrospective study, Bata et al. (2019) found that a limbal approach resulted in better visual acuity and lower complication rates compared to the pars plana approach [41]. Among 58 infants undergoing early combined LV before 7 months of age, 43% of eyes treated via limbal access achieved BCVA better than 1.0 logMAR, compared to only 11% via pars plana access [41]. Importantly, RD occurred significantly more in the latter group, highlighting the potential safety advantages of anterior access in specific cases [41].

Innovative surgical tools, such as endoscopic-assisted vitrectomy, are expanding the therapeutic armamentarium [42]. Otsubo et al. (2024) reported the utility of 23-gauge rigid endoscopes in enhancing posterior segment visualization in eyes with media opacity, enabling safer and more effective PFV stalk dissection [42]. No significant complications occurred in their series, suggesting endoscopic techniques may be particularly valuable in challenging PFV presentations [42].

Although visual prognosis in PFV is variable and often guarded, especially in eyes with posterior involvement or structural anomalies, surgical intervention can still yield meaningful functional and anatomical benefits in select cases [43]. As Soheilian M., et al. (2002) emphasized in their review of 54 eyes, visual improvement was possible in patients with anterior or combined PFV and a relatively preserved retina [43]. Surgical therapy should thus be individualized. The extent of fibrovascular proliferation, ocular morphology, patient age, and potential for amblyopia should guide decision-making [43].

Combined LV is frequently used in the surgical management of PFV, especially in cases involving both anterior and posterior segments, or when significant lens opacity or retrolental traction is present [37–43]. However, high-level comparative data are limited. While long-term visual outcomes vary, early and appropriately tailored intervention offers the best opportunity for anatomical success, cosmetic improvement, and functional vision [40].

A comparative overview of the clinical indications, anatomical and visual outcomes, and complications of combined LV across common pediatric pathologies is provided in Table 1.

Table 1. Summary of indications and outcomes for combined lensectomy and vitrectomy (LV) in pediatric pathologies.

Pediatric Condition	Indication for Combined LV	Reported Anatomic Outcome	Reported Visual Outcome	Common Complications	Key References
Congenital cataracts	1. Bilateral dense cataracts with posterior segment involvement. 2. VAO prevention. 3. Better posterior access	High rate of IOL stability; successful visual axis clearing in most cases	Mean BCVA 0.24 logMAR; poorer in children < 2 years; 14.9% with low vision	VAO, IOL pupillary capture, iris incarceration, and glaucoma	[10,13]
Ectopia lentis	1. Lens subluxation due to trauma or systemic conditions 2. Inadequate capsular support	Variable based on IOL type and fixation technique Higher rate of IOL dislocation in iris-fixation vs. scleral fixation	BCVA maintained or improved in 93.19% of eyes. Good visual outcome if no amblyopia or retinal pathology	IOL dislocation, elevated IOP, RD, endophthalmitis	[18–20]
ROP	Advanced stages (4/5) with anterior fibrovascular proliferation, retrolental fibrosis, or poor media clarity	96.3–31.3% retinal reattachment depending on stage. Better in Stage 4A than 5	Light perception or better in 64.1%; BCVA correlated poorly with anatomical outcome	Glaucoma, VAO, intraoperative/postoperative hemorrhage	[22,24,25]

Table 1. *Cont.*

Pediatric Condition	Indication for Combined LV	Reported Anatomic Outcome	Reported Visual Outcome	Common Complications	Key References
RD	Complex RDs with TRD, exudative changes, or opaque media requiring lens removal for adequate access	Variable. In some cases, anatomical reattachment required multiple surgeries	Generally poor outcomes	Glaucoma, retinal re-detachment	[35,36]
PFV	1. Significant anterior/posterior pathology 2. Cataract with retrolental membranes and stalk traction	Retinal traction relief in majority; greater axial elongation	Variable, depending on pathology extent. ~47% achieved BCVA better than 20/200; best outcomes when macula spared, and early surgery performed	Postoperative myopic shift, VAO, RD	[38,39,41]

Given the variety of IOL implantation techniques available for pediatric patients undergoing combined LV surgery, Table 2 summarizes these strategies, including their surgical contexts, associated outcomes, and common complications.

Table 2. Comparison of intraocular lens (IOL) implantation strategies in pediatric combined surgery.

IOL Technique	Surgical Indication	Patient Age Group	Visual Outcomes	Complications	Advantages	Key References
In-the-bag IOL	Congenital cataracts with adequate capsular support	Typically > 2 years	Mean BCVA ~0.24 logMAR; 85% achieved stable VA	VAO, pupillary capture, glaucoma, refractive shift	Preferred when capsular support intact; facilitates central fixation	[10,12]
Scleral-fixated IOL	Inadequate capsular support	Often > 5 years	93% maintained or improved BCVA postoperatively	IOL dislocation, elevated IOP, RD, endophthalmitis	Secure fixation without iris manipulation; avoids anterior chamber crowding	[18]
Iris-sutured IOL	Inadequate capsular support	Often > 5 years	Comparable to aphakic correction; acceptable BCVA in most patients	IOL decentration, pigment dispersion, glaucoma risk, chronic uveitis	Avoids scleral suturing; suitable when scleral fixation not possible	[20]
Aphakia (no IOL implanted)	Infants < 2 years old, or eyes with microphthalmia, severe PFV, or poor prognosis	<2 years or cases with ocular growth concerns	Limited in many cases, depending on comorbidities; amblyopia risk	VAO; glaucoma; need for secondary IOL later; rehabilitation burden	Avoids IOL complications; allows ocular growth	[39,40]

Limitations of this review include the low frequency and clinical complexity of the ocular conditions discussed, which limit the availability of robust data on this topic. Most of the included studies are retrospective and show variability in patient populations, surgical techniques, outcome measures, and follow-up durations. Additionally, many are single-center studies with small sample sizes, which may affect the generalizability of findings. Despite these limitations, this review provides a structured summary of the current literature on combined LV in pediatric patients, organized by clinical indication. It offers practical insight into when and why combined LV may be appropriate in children and highlights areas where future research is needed.

5. Conclusions

This review underscores the importance of a tailored, case-by-case surgical approach when managing pediatric patients requiring cataract extraction, lensectomy, and/or vitrectomy. While LSV is often preferred to preserve accommodation, combined LV procedures are frequently necessary in the presence of complex anterior-posterior segment pathology.

Outcomes following combined LV in children remain highly variable and are influenced by multiple factors, including patient age, underlying ocular anatomy, disease severity, and surgical technique. Although anatomic success is commonly achievable, functional visual outcomes are often limited. Moreover, combined LV is associated with a higher risk of postoperative complications such as glaucoma, VAO, and IOL dislocation, underscoring the need for long-term follow-up and comprehensive visual rehabilitation strategies.

Future studies and harmonized multicenter registries are essential to refine surgical indications and improve outcomes in this complex pediatric population. Although randomized clinical trials provide the highest level of evidence, their design and implementation in this context are challenging due to the rarity of combined LV procedures in children, the heterogeneity of underlying conditions, and the need for long-term follow-up to assess visual outcomes. However, we believe that outcome variability can be partially addressed through collaborative, prospective data collection. Rather than advocating for a universal protocol, future efforts should focus on establishing clinical principles based on shared outcome predictors such as patient age, ocular anatomy, and surgical indication. We propose the implementation of retrospective analyses using large databases such as the IRIS Registry or the Vestrum Health database. These resources could enable meaningful evaluations of surgical outcomes and complications in pediatric patients, supporting more consistent and informed decision-making while preserving individualized patient care.

Author Contributions: Conceptualization, A.J.R.-J. and V.M.V.; writing—original draft preparation, A.J.R.-J.; writing—review and editing, A.J.R.-J., V.M.V., V.C.-V., S.G.S. and T.G.M.; supervision, V.M.V., V.C.-V., S.G.S. and T.G.M. All authors have read and agreed to the published version of the manuscript.

Funding: This research received no external funding.

Conflicts of Interest: The authors declare no conflicts of interest.

References

1. Pandey, S.K.; Wilson, M.E.; Trivedi, R.H.; Izak, A.M.; Macky, T.A.; Werner, L.; Apple, D.J. Pediatric cataract surgery and intraocular lens implantation: Current techniques, complications, and management. *Int. Ophthalmol. Clin.* **2001**, *41*, 175–196. [CrossRef]
2. Medsinge, A.; Nischal, K.K. Pediatric cataract: Challenges and future directions. *Clin Ophthalmol.* **2015**, *9*, 77–90. [CrossRef]
3. Gupta, P.; Gurnani, B.; Patel, B.C. Pediatric Cataract. In *StatPearls [Internet]*; StatPearls Publishing: Treasure Island, FL, USA, 2024. Available online: https://www.ncbi.nlm.nih.gov/books/NBK572080/ (accessed on 8 June 2024).
4. Villegas, V.M.; Murray, T.G. Strategies for Combination Vitreoretinal-Cataract Surgery in Pediatric and Adult Patients. *Retin. Physician* **2017**, *14*, 32–35.
5. McDermott, M.L.; Puklin, J.E.; Abrams, G.W. Phacoemulsification for cataract following pars plana vitrectomy. *Ophthalmic Surg. Lasers* **1997**, *28*, 558–569. [CrossRef]
6. Lee, B.J.; Jun, J.H.; Afshari, N.A. Challenges and outcomes of cataract surgery after vitrectomy. *Curr. Opin. Ophthalmol.* **2025**, *36*, 70–75. [CrossRef] [PubMed]

7. Fernandez, T.A.; Carr, E.W.; Hajrasouliha, A.R. Cataract Formation Following Pars Plana Vitrectomy in the Pediatric Population. *J. Pediatr. Ophthalmol. Strabismus* **2023**, *60*, 421–426. [CrossRef]
8. Sheeladevi, S.; Lawrenson, J.G.; Fielder, A.R.; Suttle, C.M. Global prevalence of childhood cataract: A systematic review. *Eye* **2016**, *30*, 1160–1169. [CrossRef] [PubMed]
9. Esposito Veneruso, P.; Ziccardi, L.; Magli, G.; Parisi, V.; Falsini, B.; Magli, A. Developmental visual deprivation: Long term effects on human cone driven retinal function. *Graefes Arch. Clin. Exp. Ophthalmol.* **2017**, *255*, 2481–2486. [CrossRef] [PubMed]
10. Li, H.; Lin, X.; Liu, X.; Zhou, X.; Yang, T.; Fan, F.; Luo, Y. Surgical Outcomes of Lensectomy-Vitrectomy with Primary Intraocular Lens Implantation in Children with Bilateral Congenital Cataracts. *J. Pers. Med.* **2023**, *13*, 189. [CrossRef]
11. Khokhar, S.; Chandel, L.; Rani, D.; Rathod, A.; Nathiya, V.; Pujari, A. Visual axis opacification after pediatric cataract surgery—An analysis of morphology and etiology. *Indian J. Ophthalmol.* **2024**, *72* (Suppl. S4), S623–S627. [CrossRef]
12. Kugelberg, M.; Zetterström, C. Pediatric cataract surgery with or without anterior vitrectomy. *J. Cataract. Refract. Surg.* **2002**, *28*, 1770–1773. [CrossRef] [PubMed]
13. Yen, K.G.; Repka, M.X.; Sutherland, D.R.; Haider, K.M.; Hatt, S.R.; Kraker, R.T.; Galvin, J.A.; Li, Z.; Cotter, S.A.; Holmes, J.M.; et al. Complications Occurring Through 5 Years Following Primary Intraocular Lens Implantation for Pediatric Cataract. *JAMA Ophthalmol.* **2023**, *141*, 705–714. [CrossRef] [PubMed]
14. Lenhart, P.D.; Lambert, S.R. Current management of infantile cataracts. *Surv. Ophthalmol.* **2022**, *67*, 1476–1505. [CrossRef] [PubMed]
15. Vasavada, V. Paradigms for Pediatric Cataract Surgery. *Asia-Pac. J. Ophthalmol.* **2018**, *7*, 123–127. [CrossRef]
16. Neely, D.E.; Plager, D.A. Management of ectopia lentis in children. *Ophthalmol. Clin. N. Am.* **2001**, *14*, 493–499. [CrossRef] [PubMed]
17. Kaur, K.; Gurnani, B. Ectopia Lentis. In *StatPearls [Internet]*; StatPearls Publishing: Treasure Island, FL, USA, 2023. Available online: https://www.ncbi.nlm.nih.gov/books/NBK578193/ (accessed on 11 June 2023).
18. Sen, P.; S., V.K.; Bhende, P.; Rishi, P.; Rishi, E.; Rao, C.; Ratra, D.; Susvar, P.; Kummamuri, S.; Shaikh, S.; et al. Surgical outcomes and complications of sutured scleral fixated intraocular lenses in pediatric eyes. *Can. J. Ophthalmol.* **2018**, *53*, 49–55. [CrossRef]
19. Sen, P.; Shaikh, S.I.; Sreelakshmi, K. Rhegmatogenous retinal detachment in paediatric patients after pars plana vitrectomy and sutured scleral-fixated intraocular lenses. *Eye* **2018**, *32*, 345–351. [CrossRef]
20. Kopel, A.C.; Carvounis, P.E.; Hamill, M.B.; Weikert, M.P.; Holz, E.R. Iris-sutured intraocular lenses for ectopia lentis in children. *J. Cataract. Refract. Surg.* **2008**, *34*, 596–600. [CrossRef]
21. Kusaka, S. Current concepts and techniques of vitrectomy for retinopathy of prematurity. *Taiwan J. Ophthalmol.* **2018**, *8*, 216–221. [CrossRef]
22. Sen, P.; Bhende, P.; Maitra, P. Surgical outcomes in aggressive retinopathy of prematurity (AROP)-related retinal detachments. *Indian J. Ophthalmol.* **2023**, *71*, 3454–3459. [CrossRef]
23. Özsaygili, C.; Ozdek, S.; Ozmen, M.C.; Atalay, H.T.; Yalinbas Yeter, D. Parameters affecting postoperative success of surgery for stage 4A/4B ROP. *Br. J. Ophthalmol.* **2019**, *103*, 1624–1632. [CrossRef] [PubMed]
24. Chang, Y.H.; Kang, E.Y.; Chen, K.J.; Wang, N.-K.; Liu, L.; Hwang, Y.-S.; Lai, C.-C.; Wu, W.-C. Long-term surgical outcomes and prognostic factors for advanced-stage retinopathy of prematurity after vitrectomy. *Br. J. Ophthalmol.* **2024**, *109*, 126–132. [CrossRef]
25. Fei, P.; Liang, T.Y.; Peng, J.; Xu, Y.; Luo, J.; Zhang, Q.; Li, J.-K.; Lyu, J.; Zhao, P.-Q. Staged lensectomy and vitrectomy in the management of stage 5C retinopathy of prematurity with corneal opacification: Long-term follow up. *Int. J. Ophthalmol.* **2022**, *15*, 1437–1443. [CrossRef] [PubMed]
26. Chandra, P.; Kumawat, D.; Tewari, R. Hybrid clear corneal micro-incision surgical technique for stage 5 retinopathy of prematurity. *Indian J. Ophthalmol.* **2019**, *67*, 936–938. [CrossRef]
27. Chandra, P.; Tewari, R.; Salunkhe, N.; Kumawat, D.; Chaurasia, A.K.; Gupta, V. Short-term incidence and management of glaucoma after successful surgery for stage 4 retinopathy of prematurity. *Indian J. Ophthalmol.* **2019**, *67*, 917–921. [CrossRef]
28. Nudleman, E.; Muftuoglu, I.K.; Gaber, R.; Robinson, J.; Drenser, K.; Capone, A.; Trese, M.T. Glaucoma after Lens-Sparing Vitrectomy for Advanced Retinopathy of Prematurity. *Ophthalmology* **2018**, *125*, 671–675. [CrossRef] [PubMed]
29. Chehaibou, I.; Abdelmassih, Y.; Metge, F.; Chapron, T.; Dureau, P.; Caputo, G. Outcomes of Modified Limbal Lensectomy-Vitrectomy in Stages 4B and 5 Retinopathy of Prematurity with Extended Retrolental Fibroplasia. *Ophthalmol. Retin.* **2024**, *8*, 590–599. [CrossRef]
30. Rishi, E.; Srinivasan, B.; Singh, N.; Gopal, L. Late onset Descemet's membrane detachment: 15 years after limbal lensectomy with vitrectomy for ROP. *Indian J. Ophthalmol.* **2019**, *67*, 965–966. [CrossRef]
31. Bellucci, C.; Romano, A.; Ramanzini, F.; Tedesco, S.A.; Gandolfi, S.; Mora, P. Pars Plana Vitrectomy Alone or Combined with Phacoemulsification to Treat Rhegmatogenous Retinal Detachment: A Systematic Review of the Recent Literature. *J. Clin. Med.* **2023**, *12*, 5021. [CrossRef]

32. Weinberg, D.V.; Lyon, A.T.; Greenwald, M.J.; Mets, M.B. Rhegmatogenous retinal detachments in children: Risk factors and surgical outcomes. *Ophthalmology* **2003**, *110*, 1708–1713. [CrossRef]
33. Haugstad, M.; Moosmayer, S.; Bragadóttir, R. Primary rhegmatogenous retinal detachment-surgical methods and anatomical outcome. *Acta Ophthalmol.* **2017**, *95*, 247–251. [CrossRef]
34. Ferrone, P.J.; Harrison, C.; Trese, M.T. Lens clarity after lens-sparing vitrectomy in a pediatric population. *Ophthalmology* **1997**, *104*, 273–278. [CrossRef] [PubMed]
35. Mendoza, S.; Kozek, L.K.; Meng, D.; Hoyek, S.; Gonzalez, E.; Patel, N.A. Exudative retinal detachment in a pediatric patient with Rubinstein-Taybi syndrome. *Retin. Cases Brief Rep.* **2025**. [CrossRef]
36. Kawaguchi, N.; Mano, F.; Kondo, H.; Kuniyoshi, K.; Kusaka, S. Two Cases of Rubinstein-Taybi Syndrome with Retinal Detachment. *Cureus* **2025**, *17*, e80048. [CrossRef] [PubMed]
37. Loukovaara, S. Surgical Outcomes of Children with Unilateral Congenital Cataract and Persistent Fetal Vasculature. *Clin. Ophthalmol.* **2024**, *18*, 2387–2396. [CrossRef] [PubMed]
38. Lyu, J.; Zhao, P. Intraocular lens implantation in combination with lensectomy and vitrectomy for persistent fetal vasculature. *Graefes Arch. Clin. Exp. Ophthalmol.* **2020**, *258*, 2849–2856. [CrossRef]
39. Khurana, S.; Ram, J.; Singh, R.; Gupta, P.C.; Gupta, R.; Yangzes, S.; Sukhija, J.; Dogra, M.R. Surgical outcomes of cataract surgery in anterior and combined persistent fetal vasculature using a novel surgical technique: A single center, prospective study. *Graefes Arch. Clin. Exp. Ophthalmol.* **2021**, *259*, 213–221. [CrossRef]
40. Huang, H.C.; Lai, C.H.; Kang, E.Y.; Chen, K.-J.; Wang, N.-K.; Liu, L.; Hwang, Y.-S.; Lai, C.-C.; Wu, W.-C. Retrospective Analysis of Surgical Outcomes on Axial Length Elongation in Eyes with Posterior and Combined Persistent Fetal Vasculature. *Int. J. Mol. Sci.* **2023**, *24*, 5836. [CrossRef]
41. Bata, B.M.; Chiu, H.H.; Mireskandari, K.; Ali, A.; Lam, W.C.; Wan, M.J. Long-term visual and anatomic outcomes following early surgery for persistent fetal vasculature: A single-center, 20-year review. *J. AAPOS* **2019**, *23*, e1–e327. [CrossRef]
42. Otsubo, M.; Kaga, T.; Yokoyama, Y.; Kojima, T. Endoscopic Surgery for Congenital or Acquired Cataract Associated with Persistent Fetal Vasculature: A Case Series. *Retin. Cases Brief Rep.* **2024**. [CrossRef]
43. Soheilian, M.; Vistamehr, S.; Rahmani, B.; Ahmadieh, H.; Azarmina, M.; Mashayekhi, A.; Sajjadi, H.; Dehghan, M. Outcomes of surgical (pars plicata and limbal lensectomy, vitrectomy) and non-surgical management of persistent fetal vasculature (PFV): An analysis of 54 eyes. *Eur. J. Ophthalmol.* **2002**, *12*, 523–533. [CrossRef] [PubMed]

medicina

MDPI

Review

Retinitis Pigmentosa: From Genetic Insights to Innovative Therapeutic Approaches—A Literature Review

Ricardo A. Murati Calderón [1,*], Andres Emanuelli [1,2] and Natalio Izquierdo [3]

[1] Department of Ophthalmology, School of Medicine, University of Puerto Rico, San Juan 00936-5067, Puerto Rico; aemanuelli@gmail.com
[2] Emanuelli Research and Development, Retina Care, Arecibo 00612-4368, Puerto Rico
[3] Department of Surgery, University of Puerto Rico, Medical Sciences Campus, San Juan 00936-5067, Puerto Rico; njuan@msn.com
* Correspondence: ricardo.murati@upr.edu

Abstract: Retinitis pigmentosa (RP) is a heterogeneous group of inherited retinal dystrophies characterized by progressive photoreceptor degeneration and vision loss. While current management is largely supportive—relying on visual aids, orientation training, and nutritional supplementation—these interventions offer only symptomatic relief and do not halt disease progression. Advances in molecular genetics have led to the development of targeted treatments, including gene replacement therapy, RNA-based therapies, and CRISPR/Cas9 gene editing, offering promising strategies for disease modification. The approval of voretigene neparvovec for *RPE65*-associated RP marked a milestone in gene therapy, while ongoing trials targeting mutations in *RPGR*, *USH2A*, and *CEP290* are expanding therapeutic options. Optogenetic therapy and stem cell transplantation represent additional strategies, particularly for patients with advanced disease. Challenges persist in delivery efficiency, immune responses, and treating large or dominant-negative mutations. Non-viral vectors, nanoparticle systems, and artificial intelligence-guided diagnostics are being explored to address these limitations and support personalized care. This review summarizes the current and emerging therapeutic landscape for RP, highlighting the shift toward precision medicine and the need for continued innovation to overcome genetic and phenotypic variability.

Keywords: retinitis pigmentosa; genetics; inherited retinal disease; gene therapy; optogenetics; cell-based therapy; retinal prosthetics; multidisciplinary approach

1. Introduction

1.1. Overview

Retinitis pigmentosa (RP) is a group of inherited retinal dystrophies characterized by the progressive degeneration of photoreceptor cells, ultimately leading to vision loss. Patients typically experience nyctalopia initially, followed by gradual peripheral vision constriction, and in advanced stages, progress to central vision loss [1]. The prevalence of RP is estimated at approximately 1 in 4000 individuals globally [2]. Most cases are classified as non-syndromic, where retinal degeneration occurs in isolation. However, approximately 30% of RP cases are syndromic, which means that they occur in conjunction with systemic features as part of broader genetic disorders such as the Usher syndrome and Bardet–Biedl syndrome [3].

Genetically, RP is highly heterogeneous, with mutations identified in over 80 genes inherited in autosomal dominant, autosomal recessive, or X-linked patterns [1]. Mutations in genes such as *RHO* (Rhodopsin), *RP1*, and *RPGR* (retinitis pigmentosa GTPase regulator) have been among the most described, leading to a disruption in key photoreceptor functions with subsequent retinal degeneration [4,5]. *RHO* mutations are a leading cause of autosomal dominant RP (adRP), whereas *USH2A* (Usher Syndrome Type 2A) is the most frequently mutated gene in autosomal recessive RP (arRP) [6]. In contrast, mutations in *RPGR* account for most X-linked RP cases [7]. Due to the irreversible nature of photoreceptor loss, early diagnosis is crucial for optimizing disease management, allowing genetic counseling, lifestyle modifications, and the consideration of emerging therapeutic interventions to preserve vision [8]. Early disease identification is critical as many experimental therapies are mutation-specific and most effective when initiated before significant retinal damage has occurred.

1.2. Current Treatment Landscape

However, current treatment options for RP remain limited and are primarily supportive. These include low vision aids, orientation and mobility training, and nutritional supplements [9,10]. Low vision aids and orientation and mobility training help maximize residual vision and improve quality of life in patients with RP [11]. Nutritional supplements, particularly vitamin A palmitate, have been studied for their potential to slow disease progression, although the evidence remains mixed [12]. Device-based approaches, such as retinal prostheses, have also been developed to partially restore visual perception in patients with advanced RP, though accessibility and functional outcomes remain variable. Despite these interventions, existing therapies primarily address symptoms rather than the underlying genetic causes of RP. This limitation highlights the need for advanced therapeutic approaches, such as gene- and cell-based therapies, which target disease mechanisms and offer long-term solutions [13].

Recent years have witnessed transformative progress in RP therapeutics. The approval of voretigene neparvovec-rzyl (Luxturna®) for *RPE65*-associated retinal dystrophy marked a milestone in gene therapy, while ongoing clinical trials now explore gene editing (CRISPR), RNA-based correction strategies, optogenetics, and stem cell transplantation. Furthermore, the integration of artificial intelligence into molecular diagnostics and genotype–phenotype prediction is rapidly enhancing personalized care.

This review aims to synthesize the current understanding of retinitis pigmentosa from a genetic and molecular perspective while outlining the latest advancements in gene therapy, RNA-based interventions, optogenetics, and regenerative medicine. By examining the strengths and limitations of emerging therapeutic strategies, this work highlights the growing role of personalized, mutation-specific approaches in reshaping the management of RP.

2. Pathophysiology

2.1. Genetic Mutations

RP is caused by pathogenic mutations that impair critical photoreceptor cell functions. To date, more than 80 causative genes have been identified, many of which encode proteins involved in phototransduction, ciliary transport, protein folding, and visual cycle metabolism [8,14]. These include *RHO*, *RPGR*, *USH2A*, *RPE65*, and *PRPF31*, among others. Recent genotype–phenotype correlation studies emphasize that different mutations, even within the same gene, can result in distinct clinical trajectories [8].

Mutations in key genes disrupt essential photoreceptor functions, triggering a cascade of degenerative processes. For example, *RPE65* mutations impair the visual cycle by disrupting the conversion of all-trans-retinol to 11-cis-retinal, a critical process for phototransduction [15]. Similarly, *RPGR* mutations, which primarily affect ciliary transport mechanisms in photoreceptors, contribute to the progressive degeneration of both rods and cones [16]. *USH2A* mutations disrupt the structural organization of retinal photoreceptors, leading to compromised cellular integrity with progressive cell loss [17]. Mutations in *RHO*, which encode the light-sensitive rhodopsin protein in rod cells, lead to protein misfolding, endoplasmic reticulum stress, and finally to increased susceptibility to photoreceptor apoptosis [18].

Collectively, these mutations impair essential photoreceptor functions, leading to metabolic imbalance, oxidative stress, and the activation of proinflammatory and apoptotic pathways, ultimately culminating in photoreceptor cell death.

2.2. *Mechanisms of Retinal Degeneration*

The effects of mutations initiate a cascade of degenerative processes in the retina, which follows a series of interrelated mechanisms primarily driven by photoreceptor cell apoptosis. Rod cells, with their high metabolic demands and oxygen consumption, are especially susceptible to the oxidative stress caused by the production of reactive oxygen species (ROS)—a byproduct of their intense aerobic metabolism [19]. As rod cells degenerate, the oxygen demand in the retina decreases, leading to increased levels of local oxygen, a condition known as retinal hyperoxia. This excess oxygen in the retina promotes the production of ROS, which increases oxidative damage to the remaining photoreceptors and retinal pigment epithelial (RPE) cells [20]. This secondary degeneration of retinal photoreceptors caused by the excessive oxidative stress from initial rod cell death, despite direct genetic defects, has been described as the bystander effect and is a hallmark of RP progression [21].

Inflammatory responses also play a key role in the pathogenesis of RP. The degeneration of photoreceptors triggers microglial activation--the primary immune cells of the retina—which release proinflammatory cytokines, leading to chronic inflammation and exacerbating retinal damage [22]. In addition, dysregulated microglial phagocytic activity has been described, contributing to the excessive clearance of stressed photoreceptors and promoting further neuronal loss. Worsening the degenerative cascade, the accumulation of misfolded proteins due to genetic mutations activates intracellular stress pathways, notably the unfolded protein response (UPR), which further drives photoreceptor apoptosis [18].

2.3. *Genetic Heterogeneity*

The clinical presentation of RP varies significantly based on the underlying genetic mutation and inheritance pattern. Autosomal dominant RP (AdRP), typically associated with *RHO* mutations, generally progresses more slowly than autosomal recessive RP (arRP). The latter results from loss-of-function gene mutations such as *USH2A* and *RPE65* [4]. X-linked RP, often linked to *RPGR* mutations, is one of the most severe forms, with the early onset and rapid progression of the disease [23]. The identification of the gene and its inheritance pattern helps predict the phenotypic expression and prognosis of the disease. Furthermore, it underscores the clinical heterogeneity in patients with RP due to various gene mutations.

Recent studies suggest that modifier genes, epigenetic factors, and environmental influences can further modulate disease severity. For example, patients with identical mutations may have varying degrees of photoreceptor dysfunction, suggesting that additional genetic and non-genetic factors contribute to disease progression [24–26].

3. Genetic Therapy Strategies

Understanding the complex genetic framework is essential for developing targeted and personalized treatment strategies. In recent decades, advancements in molecular genetics and retinal biology have transformed the therapeutic view for retinitis pigmentosa. As traditional interventions primarily offer symptomatic relief or the subtle preservation of visual function, they fail to address the root genetic causes driving photoreceptor degeneration. With the identification of specific pathogenic mutations and a deeper understanding of disease mechanisms, gene-based therapies have emerged as a promising tool for targeted intervention. These novel strategies aim to slow disease progression and restore visual function by correcting for the underlying genetic defects. We will explore the major categories of genetic therapies currently under investigation or in clinical use for RP.

3.1. Gene Replacement Therapy

Gene replacement therapy aims to restore retinal function by delivering copies of genes into retinal cells harboring pathogenic mutations, typically using viral vectors. One of the most notable clinical applications is voretigene neparvovec-rzyl (Luxturna®), the first FDA-approved gene therapy for an inherited retinal disease. Luxturna uses an adeno-associated viral (AAV) vector–mediated therapy for *RPE65*-associated retinal dystrophy [27].

In the phase 3 clinical trial, 29 patients with *RPE65*-associated retinal dystrophy received subretinal injections of Luxturna. At 1-year post-treatment, 65% of participants demonstrated clinical improvement in functional vision, as assessed by the multi-luminance mobility test (MLMT), compared to only 10% in the control group. Additionally, full-field light sensitivity threshold (FST) and BCVA revealed improvements with effects sustained through long-term follow-ups, with some seen for up to 4 years. Ultimately, no serious adverse events related to the gene product were reported, confirming a favorable safety profile [27,28]. After Luxturna's success, multiple ongoing clinical trials have explored gene replacement approaches for other RP-related mutations. For instance, a phase 1/2 in-human clinical trial evaluated an AAV-based vector encoding an optimized *RPGR* gene in patients with X-linked RP. Preliminary results at 6 months demonstrated preserved retinal structure and visual function with no dosage-associated limiting toxicities [29]. These efforts suggest gene replacement therapy as a promising viable treatment option for specific RP subtypes.

Despite these successes, challenges persist in optimizing gene delivery to the retina. The complex structural organization of the retina complicates vector penetration and limits efficient transduction. For example, subretinal injection allows direct delivery to photoreceptors and RPE cells but is invasive and carries the risk of retinal detachment and inflammation. In contrast, despite being less invasive with decreased risks, intravitreal injection often results in low transduction efficiency due to dilution in the vitreous and the potential immune responses within the vitreous [30]. Furthermore, AAV vectors have a limited packaging capacity, restricting their use in diseases caused by mutations in large genes [31]. This capacity represents a significant challenge when targeting genes with large coding sequences, such as *IFT140*, *USH2A*, and *EYS*, all implicated in various forms of RP.

A further challenge in AAV-mediated gene delivery for RP arises from pre-existing immunity. Humans are naturally exposed to wild-type AAV serotypes, particularly AAV2, resulting in neutralizing antibodies that may interfere with vector efficacy. This is especially relevant for intravitreal administration, where the vector is more likely to interact with immune components in the vitreous. In contrast, subretinal delivery offers partial immune privilege by limiting systemic exposure. Nevertheless, serotype selection remains critical. Several ongoing trials utilize engineered or less prevalent serotypes (e.g., AAV8, AAV9) to enhance transduction efficiency and reduce the risk of immune neutralization. Strategies such as immune screening before treatment and immunomodulatory regimens are also under investigation to address this barrier in gene therapy for inherited retinal diseases [31].

In addition to immune neutralization, AAV-based gene therapies have raised safety concerns related to potential liver toxicity, particularly with systemic or high-dose administration. Although ocular gene delivery is largely localized, minimizing systemic exposure, recent reports have identified hepatotoxic effects in some AAV serotypes under different delivery contexts. While such risks are reduced in the subretinal delivery used in RP trials, caution remains warranted, especially as novel serotypes and delivery routes are explored [31].

Multi-vector recombination strategies have been studied to address the limited packaging capacity. For example, Datta and co-workers implemented a recombination system using the CRE-lox system to deliver the large *IFT140* gene [32]. The approach utilized up to four AAV vectors, each encoding fragments of the therapeutic gene. The strategy successfully reconstituted the full-length *ITF140* in cultured mammalian cells and mouse retinas. Importantly, when dual AAV vectors delivering the *IFT140* gene were administered in the sub-retinal space in a conditional knockout mouse model, the therapy significantly preserved the photoreceptor structure, maintained retinal function (measured via ERG response), and prevented retinal degeneration [32]. While these findings demonstrate promising preclinical efficacy, the Cre-lox system presents translational challenges for human therapy. These include concerns about recombination efficiency in human retinal tissue, vector packaging complexity, and regulatory hurdles related to the co-administration of multiple viral vectors. Additional studies are needed to optimize recombination fidelity, assess immunogenicity, and evaluate the safety profile in large-animal models before considering clinical application.

Another innovative approach involves the use of split intein-mediated protein trans-splicing. This method allows for the delivery of large genes by splitting them into smaller fragments that can be packaged into separate AAV vectors. For example, Tornabene and co-workers demonstrated the successful expression of full-length *ABCA4* and *CEP290* in mouse and pig retinas [33]. Despite these challenges, ongoing innovations in vector design, delivery techniques, and immune modulation are steadily improving the safety and effectiveness of retinal gene therapy.

3.2. Gene Editing Approaches

Gene editing approaches are promising for treating patients with RP by correcting deleterious mutations at the DNA level [34]. Among these, the Clustered Regularly Interspaced Short Palindromic Repeats/CRISPR-associated protein 9 (CRISPR/Cas9) is a gene-editing system derived from bacterial adaptive immunity that enables site-specific DNA cleavage and repair through the guidance of RNA molecules [35]. This technology allows one to make precise modifications to the genome, restoring normal gene function and halting disease progression [34]. A landmark example is EDIT-101, a CRISPR/Cas9 gene-editing complex targeting the *CEP290* gene. In the phase 1/2 BRILLIANCE clinical trial, Pierce and co-workers reported that 43% of patients who received EDIT-101 demonstrated a visually meaningful improvement in retinal sensitivity, with additional gains observed in BCVA and quality-of-life measures [36]. Preclinical studies have shown that CRISPR/Cas9 can effectively target and correct gene mutations such as *RPGR*, leading to photoreceptor preservation and functional improvement in mouse models. Notably, no detectable off-target editing effects, where unintended DNA regions may be altered, were reported for up to 12 months following treatment [37].

However, despite these promising results in gene editing, several ethical considerations should be addressed. The potential unintended genetic modifications raise safety concerns. Also, long-term monitoring is essential to ensure that gene editing does not introduce further deleterious mutations or trigger immune responses [38].

3.3. RNA-Based Therapies

RNA-based therapies offer alternative strategies for treating patients with RP by targeting mutant mRNA transcripts. Antisense oligonucleotides (AONs) are short, single-stranded DNA or RNA molecules that specifically bind to complementary sequences on target pre-mRNA. Hence, AONs can modulate RNA processing in several ways, notably by blocking access to splice sites. In the context of RP, AONs are particularly useful in correcting aberrant splicing events caused by intronic or exomic mutations, ultimately restoring the open reading frame and enabling the translation of a functional protein [39].

For example, Grainok and co-workers described an AON-based exon-skipping strategy to treat RP, specifically RP11, which truncated the mutations of the pre-mRNA processing factor 31 (*PRPF31*) gene [40]. The study demonstrated that AONs could induce the selective skipping of the mutated exon, restoring the gene's open reading frame and enhancing the production of functional PRPF31 protein [40]. Similarly, research by Slijkerman and co-workers explored the use of AONs to address a deep-intronic mutation in the *USH2A* gene, which leads to the inclusion of a pseudoexon and results in a truncated, non-functional usherin protein [41]. Their work demonstrated that AON-mediated splice correction can prevent the incorporation of the pseudoexon, thereby restoring regular usherin protein expression and function [41]. Both these studies highlight the therapeutic potential of AONs in RP by precisely manipulating mRNA splicing events to overcome the effects of deleterious mutations.

While complementing the splice-modifying capacities of AONs, RNA interference (RNAi) offers a distinct mechanism of action by selectively silencing mutant gene transcripts. This process is mediated by small interfering RNAs (siRNAs) or short hairpin RNAs (shRNAs), which are designed to specifically bind complementary sequences within the target mRNA, leading to its cleavage and preventing translation into dysfunctional proteins. Specifically, Guzman-Aranguez and co-workers reviewed several RNAi-based strategies targeting retinal diseases, highlighting the therapeutic potential of siRNAs in RP by silencing pathogenic rhodopsin transcripts [42]. O'Reilly and co-workers demonstrated the suppression of mutant rhodopsin (*RHO*) transcripts via the application of RNAi in patients with autosomal dominant RP. The study showed that RNAi can have up to a 90% suppression of *RHO* expression in photoreceptors using AAV vectors for delivery [43]. Therefore, these studies underscore the potential of RNA-based therapies in RP, offering a targeted approach to mitigate photoreceptor degeneration and preserve visual function.

While both gene editing and RNA-based therapies offer targeted treatment strategies for RP, they differ significantly in mechanism, durability, and clinical considerations. Gene editing approaches such as CRISPR/Cas9 aim to permanently correct pathogenic DNA mutations through a single intervention, potentially offering long-term or curative benefit. However, safety concerns, particularly related to off-target editing, immunogenicity, and long-term genomic stability, require ongoing monitoring and ethical caution. In contrast, RNA-based therapies like AONs and RNAi modulate gene expression at the transcript level and are generally well tolerated. Their transient nature typically necessitates repeated administration to maintain efficacy but reduces the risk of permanent genomic alteration. From a cost perspective, RNA-based strategies may offer more accessible short-term interventions, whereas gene editing, although more resource-intensive, holds promise for durable, mutation-specific treatment. Together, these approaches represent complementary strategies in the evolving landscape of personalized retinal therapeutics.

3.4. Optogenetic Therapy

In contrast to therapies that aim to correct or silence genetic defects, optogenetic therapy offers a novel approach by re-engineering light sensitivity in retinal cells downstream of the photoreceptors. This modality is used for patients with advanced RP, particularly those with extensive photoreceptor loss [44]. This strategy involves introducing genes that encode light-sensitive proteins—such as channel-rhodopsins—into surviving inner retinal neurons, including bipolar or ganglion cells, to confer light responsiveness in the absence of functional photoreceptors [45]. By reactivating these downstream neurons, optogenetics bypasses damaged photoreceptors and creates a new photosensitive pathway [46].

In a clinical case, Sahel and colleagues reported partial visual recovery in a blind RP patient using an optogenetic construct (ChrimsonR) delivered via intravitreal injection, combined with engineered goggles that amplified and converted light into specific wavelengths, demonstrating proof-of-concept for human use [46]. Notably, no reported adverse ocular events over 84 weeks of follow-up were described. Similarly, Lindner and co-workers reviewed multiple preclinical studies where optogenetic tools successfully activated retinal ganglion cells in RP animal models, restoring light responses and allowing basic visual behaviors [46].

The RESTORE trial, a Phase 2b randomized, double-masked, sham-controlled study conducted by Nanoscope Therapeutics, evaluated the efficacy of MCO-010, an ambient light-activatable multi-characteristic opsin (MCO) gene therapy for patients with advanced retinitis pigmentosa. The therapy, delivered via intravitreal injection, demonstrated statistically significant improvements in visual function in preclinical models of retinitis pigmentosa. Treated mice exhibited enhanced optomotor responses, faster spatial navigation in visually guided water-maze tests, and improved visually evoked potentials compared to the controls. These functional gains persisted for up to 26 weeks post-injection. Importantly, MCO-010 was well tolerated, with no evidence of ocular toxicity, phototoxicity, or systemic immunogenicity. These results underscore the potential of optogenetic therapy as a gene-agnostic treatment strategy for patients with late-stage RP [47].

While promising, optogenetic therapy is currently limited by the need for external light amplification devices, restricted spatial resolution, and dependence on viable inner retinal circuits. Nonetheless, this approach holds significant potential for patients in the late stages of RP, where traditional photoreceptor-targeted therapies are no longer viable.

Table 1 summarizes the primary gene-based therapeutic strategies currently explored in retinitis pigmentosa, detailing their mechanisms of action, delivery methods, outcomes, and limitations in clinical and preclinical settings.

Table 1. Summary of gene-based therapeutic strategies in RP.

Therapy Strategy	Mechanism/Target	Delivery Method	Recent Outcomes	Limitations
Gene Replacement Therapy	AAV-delivered gene copies to restore function (e.g., *RPE65*, *RPGR*); dual/multi-vector recombination for large genes (e.g., *IFT140*)	Subretinal injection (AAV2); dual vectors for large genes	Luxturna®: 65% improved MLMT at 1 year; *RPGR* trials show structural/functional preservation; *IFT140* dual AAV preserved function in mice	AAV packaging limits; subretinal surgery risks (detachment, inflammation)
Gene Editing (CRISPR-Cas9)	DNA-level correction (e.g., *CEP290*, *RPGR*) via RNA-guided Cas9 to restore gene function	Subretinal delivery of CRISPR complexes via viral or non-viral systems	EDIT-101: 43% showed improved retinal sensitivity; RPGR editing in mice preserved photoreceptors without off-target effects	Risk of off-target edits; ethical/safety concerns; need for long-term monitoring

Table 1. *Cont.*

Therapy Strategy	Mechanism/Target	Delivery Method	Recent Outcomes	Limitations
RNA-Based Therapies (AON, RNAi)	AONs modify splicing (e.g., *PRPF31*, *USH2A*); siRNA/shRNA silence toxic mRNA (e.g., *RHO*)	Intravitreal injection of synthetic oligos or viral-delivered RNA tools	AONs corrected splicing in *PRPF31* and *USH2A* models; RNAi achieved 90% *RHO* transcript suppression in photoreceptors	Transient effects; limited delivery efficiency; immune response potential
Optogenetic Therapy	Introduces light-sensitive opsins (e.g., ChrimsonR, MCO-010) into bipolar/ganglion cells to bypass lost photoreceptors	Intravitreal injection of gene constructs (no viable photoreceptors needed)	RESTORE trial: mice showed improved optomotor and water-maze behavior; human case regained partial vision using ChrimsonR with engineered goggles; well tolerated	Low spatial resolution; dependent on assistive devices; requires intact downstream retinal circuitry

4. Challenges in Genetic Therapy

4.1. Delivery Mechanisms

Despite genetic therapies' promising potential for RP, several challenges must be addressed to ensure their long-term safety, efficacy, and accessibility. One primary limitation involves the delivery of therapeutic genes to retinal cells.

Viral vectors, most commonly adeno-associated viruses (AAVs), are the leading medium for gene delivery due to their natural affinity for retinal cells, known as tropism, and safety profile [27]. However, AAVs have a limited carrying capacity (<5 kb), making them unsuitable for larger genes. This constraint renders AAV vectors unsuitable for delivering large genes, including *USH2A*, *EYS*, or *ABCA4*, which exceed this size threshold [33,48]. For example, Trapani and co-workers emphasized that approximately one-third of genes implicated in inherited retinal diseases exceed the natural capacity of AAV vectors, presenting an obstacle to therapeutic development [49]. Their review study highlighted that an attempt to compress larger cDNAs into a single AAV resulted in unstable products, leading to reduced transduction efficiency and inconsistent therapeutic expression. Similarly, Toms and co-workers noted that the full-length *USH2A* was three times the supposedly accommodated size, hence proposing the necessity for alternative strategies for effective gene delivery [48].

Physical and anatomical barriers within the eye also significantly limit AAV-mediated transduction, particularly when vectors are delivered intravitreally. Dalkara and co-workers demonstrated that the inner limiting membrane (ILM) acts as a barrier to AAV penetration, limiting gene expression in the inner retina [50]. Specifically, the study found that the co-administration of a protease to digest the ILM enabled the specific AAV serotype to transduce multiple retinal layers, an effect not previously achieved via intravitreal delivery. Subretinal injection, though effective in bypassing the ILM, is invasive and carries surgical risks such as retinal detachments [51]. In their study involving non-human primates, Gamlin and co-workers observed procedures leading to localized retinal damage. They proposed that the meticulous control during injected delivery is required to prevent iatrogenic trauma [51]. Therefore, modern subretinal injections are now guided by OCT imaging to improve safety and accuracy, allowing clinicians to monitor needle positioning during the procedure.

Beyond delivery efficiency, safety concerns such as immune responses to the viral capsid or gene product pose further obstacles. Bucher and co-workers demonstrated that these immune responses could lead to inflammation and reduced therapeutic durability, particularly in the context of adeno-associated virus (AAV) vectors used for gene therapy [31]. They showed that AAV vectors can activate Toll-like receptors (TLR), resulting in the release of inflammatory cytokines and interferons. Additionally, AAV vectors can induce capsid-specific and transgene-specific T-cell responses and anti-AAV antibodies, which limit therapeutic effects by destroying targeted cells [31].

4.2. Long-Term Efficacy and Safety

Another consideration is the sustainability of therapeutic effects over time. Although early clinical trials have shown encouraging results, long-term data on gene therapy durability is still limited. Maguire and co-workers reported that the therapeutic effects of voretigene neparvovec-rzyl (Luxturna®) were maintained for up to four years in patients with *RPE65*-associated retinal dystrophy [52]. However, Chao and co-workers also noted instances of visual function decline in some patients [53]. Concerns remain regarding gene expression stability, progressive retinal remodeling, and the potential for delayed adverse effects. As such, long-term follow-up and robust post-treatment monitoring will be essential to ensure efficacy and safety across diverse patient populations.

4.3. Personalized Medicine and Genetic Variability

Finally, the considerable genetic and phenotypic heterogeneity of RP presents challenges for personalized treatment strategies. With over 3000 mutations identified across more than 70 genes, therapies must be tailored to individual genotypes, requiring accessible and comprehensive genetic testing alongside mutation-specific delivery platforms. As highlighted by Dias and co-workers, this genetic heterogeneity necessitates the development of genotype-specific therapies and broad access to diagnostic testing to improve patient selection and clinical outcomes [12]. Similarly, Nguyen and co-workers emphasized the essential role of genetic testing not only for accurate diagnosis but also for determining the eligibility for mutation-specific therapies and advancing enrollment in appropriate clinical trials [54].

Gene replacement therapy is considered most effective in cases where the underlying mutation results in a loss of gene function and the therapeutic gene is small enough to fit within the packaging limits of vectors. As noted by Arbabi and co-workers, this approach is particularly applicable for patients with autosomal recessive RP, where biallelic loss-of-function mutations result in the absence of functional proteins [55]. Similarly, Dias and co-workers highlight that gene augmentation strategies are appropriate when the defective gene can be replaced with a functional copy [12]. However, both studies underscore the limitation regarding the packaging capacity of specific vectors such as AAVs.

In contrast, RNA-based therapies or gene editing may be more appropriate, especially when dominant-negative or splicing mutations are involved. For example, antisense oligonucleotides can modulate splicing defects, while gene editing technologies like CRISPR/Cas9 can correct specific mutations at the DNA level [40,56]. Therefore, accurate genetic diagnosis is essential to determine eligibility for targeted clinical trials or mutation-specific interventions.

Moreover, treatment response can vary significantly based on disease stage, retinal health, and individual genetic modifiers, even among patients with the same mutation [8,24,57]. These facts highlight the importance of developing therapeutic platforms that can accommodate interindividual variability, such as genetic testing, clinical profiling, and biomarker identification. Personalized approaches will be critical in advancing equitable and effective care for individuals living with RP.

Table 2 summarizes the major challenges encountered in the application of genetic therapy for RP, highlighting both the limitations and emerging solutions.

Table 2. Challenges in genetic therapy for RP.

Challenge	Advantage/Opportunity	Limitation	Proposed Solutions
Delivery Barriers	Subretinal injection allows precise targeting; capsid engineering improves vector spread	Invasive procedure; risk of detachment or inflammation; intravitreal injection has low efficiency	Use of suprachoroidal delivery, capsid optimization, and hybrid delivery systems
Vector Capacity Limitations	Gene editing and RNA-based therapies allow payload minimization	AAVs cannot carry large genes (e.g., *USH2A*, *ABCA4*)	Dual/multi-vector approaches, split-intein recombination, or alternative vectors
Immune Responses	Novel serotypes and immune modulation strategies enhance tolerability	Vector-induced immune activation may limit expression or cause inflammation	Pre-treatment with immunosuppressants, vector engineering, and monitoring biomarkers
Gene and Mutation Specificity	Precision medicine enables mutation-matched therapy	Rare variants may be untargetable or underrepresented in clinical research	Integrate gene-agnostic methods (e.g., optogenetics); develop mutation-agnostic delivery platforms
Long-Term Expression and Safety	Episomal vectors reduce genomic integration; regulatory elements can fine-tune expression	Concerns about sustained expression, gene silencing, or unforeseen effects	Use of biodegradable vectors, inducible promoters, and long-term clinical surveillance
Ethical and Regulatory Concerns	Global consensus growing around clinical gene therapy governance	Issues around germline editing, patient autonomy, and equitable access	Clear ethical oversight, patient engagement, transparent consent processes, and international policy alignment

5. Recent Advances and Clinical Trials

5.1. Overview of Key Clinical Trials

Currently, gene therapy is considered a promising treatment option for patients with RP, particularly those with biallelic *RPE65* mutations. The approval of Luxturna marked a milestone in ocular gene therapy, offering the first FDA-approved gene therapy for inherited retinal disease. In a phase 3 clinical trial, Russell et al. demonstrated significant improvements in functional vision, with 72% of patients (21 of 29) achieving successful performance on the MLMT at the lowest light level (1 lux) one-year post-treatment, compared to none achieved at baseline [28]. These results were supported by Maguire and co-workers, who demonstrated gains in light sensitivity, with mean improvements in full-field light sensitivity threshold (FST) of −2.04 log10 (cd·s/m) sustained through 3 years of follow-up [58], that is, more than 100-fold enhancement in light sensitivity.

Furthermore, visual field expansion and stability in visual acuity were also observed. For example, at 4-year follow-ups, Maguire and co-workers described patients in the original intervention group with a mean increase of 197.7 degrees in Goldmann visual field and maintained near-baseline visual acuity [58]. Similarly, in another study by Maguire, the group confirmed the long-term durability of these effects, noting that the gains in FST and MLMT performance were preserved for up to 4 years, with no serious adverse events reported, affirming the favorable safety profile of Luxturna® [52]. In some instances, adverse effects were mild and mostly attributed to the subretinal surgical procedure rather than the vector itself [52]. Hence, these results from clinical trials provide evidence that gene replacement therapy with voretigene neparvovec leads to sustained improvements in vision-related function.

Beyond *RPE65*, gene therapy trials are now expanding to address other RP genotypes. A phase I/II clinical trial (XIRIUS) targeting *RPGR*-related X-linked RP demonstrated encouraging early results. Cehajic-Kapetanovic and co-workers reported that patients receiving mid-range doses of an AAV vector to deliver codon optimized version of *RPGR* exhibited gains in retinal sensitivity and the partial reversal of visual field loss as early as 1 month, with sustained effects at 6 months [29]. However, in higher dose cohorts, cases of mild subretinal inflammation were reported.

Additionally, Pierce and co-workers evaluated EDIT-101, the first in vivo CRISPR/Cas9-based gene-editing therapy, in patients with *CEP290*-associated Leber Congenital Amaurosis (LCA10) [36]. Although LCA10 is not a form of RP, the BRILLIANCE trial represents a significant proof-of-concept for CRISPR in the retina. The study found that 64% of patients had a clinically meaningful improvement in at least one visual outcome (e.g., FST, best-corrected visual acuity, or mobility test), with no dose-limiting toxicities or serious adverse events attributed to the treatment [36]. Although still in early phases, preclinical studies have demonstrated that gene editing approaches targeting *RPGR*, including CRISPR-mediated frame restoration in ORF15, can successfully rescue photoreceptor structure and function in RP models [29,59,60]. These findings collectively underscore the therapeutic potential of gene editing platforms in inherited retinal diseases and provide a way for broader applications across RP genotypes.

Other ongoing trials are exploring gene editing technologies, such as CRISPR/Cas9, to correct mutations in genes like *CEP290* and *RPGR*, with early-stage research showing promising results in preclinical and clinical settings. For instance, a Phase 1/2 clinical trial (BRILLIANCE) is evaluating the safety and efficacy of EDIT-101, a CRISPR/Cas9-based therapy targeting the *CEP290* mutation associated with Leber Congenital Amaurosis 10 (LCA10). Although LCA10 is not a subtype of RP, the trial is significant as it represents the first clinical application of CRISPR in the retina, demonstrating in vivo gene editing. Initial findings have demonstrated favorable safety outcomes and preliminary evidence of improvements in full-field stimulus testing (FST) and best-corrected visual acuity (BCVA) in some treated patients [36].

5.2. AI-Driven Precision Medicine and Retinal Prosthetics

The integration of artificial intelligence (AI) and machine learning in RP research has the potential to revolutionize the identification of candidate genes and the optimization of therapies. These technologies enable the analysis of large-scale genetic and clinical datasets, allowing for the classification of inherited retinal diseases (IRDs), the prediction of causative genes, and disease prognosis. A study by Esteban-Medina and co-workers used machine learning to generate a mechanistic functional map of RP, identifying 226 functional circuits and predicting 109 targets of approved drugs with potential effects [61]. Some of these targets were validated in a murine model, highlighting the potential of AI-driven approaches for drug repurposing and novel therapeutic discovery [61]. Additionally, Gomes and Ashley highlighted the application of AI in molecular medicine, emphasizing its role in variant prioritization for rare diseases [62]. This ability is crucial for RP, where over 70 genes have been implicated. Fujinami-Yokokawa and co-workers demonstrated that deep learning models trained on fundus photographs and fundus autofluorescence images could predict causative IRD genes such as *EYS*, *ABCA4*, and *RP1L1* with test accuracies of up to 88.2% and specificities exceeding 95%, illustrating AI's potential to enhance non-invasive diagnostic precision in RP [63]. Similarly, Issa and co-workers noted that AI models applied to retinal imaging were able to discriminate RP images from normal images with a value of area under the receiver operating curve (AUROC) of 96.74% [64].

By leveraging machine learning algorithms, researchers and clinicians can uncover novel genetic associations and lead treatment strategies tailored to individual genetic profiles. The AI-driven methodologies are pivotal in advancing precision medicine for RP, enabling tailored interventions based on individual genetic profiles and optimizing patient outcomes.

Concurrently, advances in retinal prosthetics are expanding the treatment landscape for blind patients with RP. Retinal prosthetic devices such as epiretinal and subretinal implants aim to restore partial vision by stimulating surviving retinal neurons [65]. Clinical trials have demonstrated their potential in restoring visual perception to profoundly blind patients with RP. For example, Ho and co-workers underwent the extensive clinical evaluation of the Argus II Retinal Prothesis System, an epiretinal device [66]. The study involving 30 subjects reported an acceptable safety profile and functional benefit, with the longest implant duration reportedly reaching 7.2 years [66].

5.3. Cell-Based Therapies

Cell-based therapies may be used for RP by targeting the underlying degeneration of photoreceptors and retinal pigment epithelium (RPE) cells. These therapies aim to replace damaged retinal cells through the transplantation of stem cell-derived photoreceptors or RPE cells, potentially restoring retinal structure and function.

Preclinical studies have demonstrated that retinal progenitor cells (RPCs) can survive, integrate into the host retina, and promote photoreceptor preservation in degenerative models. Wang and co-workers reported that transplanted RPCs in rodent models of RP led to improvements in visual function and the structural integrity of the outer retina [67]. Early-phase clinical trials have also provided encouraging results. In a systematic review and meta-analysis, Chen and co-workers analyzed 21 prospective studies involving 496 eyes and found that 49% of RP patients experienced an improvement in best-corrected visual acuity (BCVA) at 6 months, although long-term benefits beyond 12 months were less significant [68]. The analysis further highlighted that suprachoroidal space injection showed the most significant BCVA improvement, suggesting it as a delivery route. Additionally, Liu and co-workers demonstrated the long-term safety and feasibility of human fetal-derived RPC transplantation in RP patients, with five out of eight patients showing improved visual acuity and three exhibiting enhanced retinal sensitivity as measured by pupillary light reflex within the first 6 months post treatment, without evidence of immune rejection or tumor formation over a two-year follow-up period [69]. These findings underscore the regenerative potential and safety profile of stem cell-based strategies in inherited retinal degenerations.

However, these technologies face several challenges. For retinal prostheses, limitations include low spatial resolution, complex surgical implantation, and limited patient adaptability. In stem cell therapies, concerns persist regarding long-term graft survival, immune rejection, and the theoretical risk of tumorigenesis. These factors highlight the need for the continued long-term evaluation of safety and efficacy in clinical trials.

Table 3 summarizes key clinical trials and emerging technological strategies in the treatment of RP, providing an overview of the therapeutic indications, major findings, and translational limitations across gene therapy, gene editing, artificial intelligence, and regenerative platforms.

Table 3. Summary of notable clinical trials and emerging technologies in RP.

Intervention/Technology	Target/Indication	Key Clinical Findings	Limitations/Considerations
Luxturna® (voretigene neparvovec)	*RPE65*-associated RP	72% MLMT success at 1 lux; FST gain −2.04 log10 cd·s/m; sustained visual field and acuity improvements for 4+ years	Requires subretinal surgery; gene-specific; not generalizable to all RP genotypes
RPGR Gene Therapy (XIRIUS trial)	X-linked RP (*RPGR* mutations)	Improved retinal sensitivity and partial visual field reversal in mid-dose groups; benefits observed as early as 1 month, sustained at 6 months	Mild subretinal inflammation at higher doses; limited to *RPGR* mutations
EDIT-101 (BRILLIANCE trial)	*CEP290* mutation (LCA10—CRISPR/Cas9 gene editing)	64% had improvements in ≥1 visual function outcome (FST, BCVA, mobility); no serious adverse events	Still in early phases; LCA10 not classified as RP but establishes retinal CRISPR precedent
AI Applications in RP	Gene identification, diagnosis, prognosis	Predicted causative genes (e.g., *EYS*, *RP1L1*) with 88.2% accuracy; AUROC 96.74% in retinal image-based classification	Not a therapy; dependent on algorithm quality, training data, and clinical integration
Argus II Retinal Prosthesis System	Advanced RP with profound vision loss	Clinical safety and functional benefit in 30 patients; device longevity up to 7.2 years	Low visual resolution; surgical implantation complexity; limited adaptability
Stem Cell Therapy (e.g., RPCs via Suprachoroidal Delivery)	RP with photoreceptor/RPE degeneration	49% of eyes showed BCVA improvement at 6 months (n = 496); best results with suprachoroidal delivery; no rejection/tumors in long-term follow-up trials	Outcomes vary by protocol; long-term efficacy unclear; risk of immune rejection and graft survival limitations

6. Future Directions and Perspectives

As the field of RP therapy continues to evolve, future directions are increasingly centered on overcoming the current limitations of gene delivery and maximizing therapeutic efficacy through multimodal approaches. To address these gaps, ongoing research is exploring next-generation delivery systems, including advanced viral vectors, nanoparticles, and non-viral platforms, aimed at improving safety, precision, and accessibility. In parallel, the integration of gene therapy with complementary modalities such as stem cell transplantation and retinal prosthetics is gaining attention as a strategy to enhance outcomes and expand the therapeutic options for individuals with advanced or genetically complex diseases.

6.1. Improving Delivery Systems

Effective delivery of therapeutic agents to retinal cells is crucial for the success of gene therapies in RP. Traditional methods, such as subretinal injections using AAV vectors, have shown promise but come with limitations, including surgical risks and limited retinal coverage. Recent innovations that aim to address these challenges include intravitreal AAV vector delivery, nanoparticle technology, and non-viral delivery systems.

ViGeneron has recently launched a clinical trial utilizing their proprietary vgAAV vector for the intravitreal delivery of the *CNGA1* gene, targeting the RP caused by *CNGA1* mutations. Prior studies have demonstrated the potential of variant AAV capsids for efficient intravitreal gene delivery to photoreceptors, crucial for treating inherited retinal diseases. For example, Pavlou and coworkers reported the development of engineered AAV vectors that enable the efficient targeting of photoreceptors via intravitreal administration [70]. In different animal models, the novel variants showed an up to 100-fold higher photoreceptor transduction efficiency compared to the unmodified AAV2 vector—a version widely used in early gene therapy research and clinical trials [70].

Additionally, He and co-workers identified a novel AAV2 capsid variant that demonstrated key improvements in treated mice, supporting its clinical potential [71]. Specifically, the intravitreal administration of the variant capsid carrying the affected gene led to significantly restored visual function, as evidenced by improved pupillary light reflex and behavioral performance in light/dark box and visual cliff tests. Similarly, through histological analysis, the authors revealed that treated mice had a preserved outer nuclear layer (ONL) thickness and significantly increased expression of the affected gene product compared to those receiving standard AAV2 vectors [71]. These two examples further support the current direction towards improving vector design.

Nanoparticle-based delivery systems, such as mesoporous silica-based nanoparticles, polymeric nanoparticles, lipid nanoparticles, and other non-viral vectors, are emerging as a promising alternative to traditional viral vectors for gene therapy in RP. These offer advantages over traditional viral vectors, such as higher safety profiles, low immunogenicity, and the capacity to deliver larger genetic payloads. In a study by Valdés-Sanchez and co-workers, mesoporous silica nanoparticles (MSNs) mediated the successful delivery of therapeutic genes to retinal cells in vivo without disrupting retinal morphology or function, as confirmed through multimodal imaging and electroretinographic studies [72]. Similarly, Maya-Vetencourt and co-workers demonstrated that conjugated polymer nanoparticles such as poly(3-hexylthiophene) (P3HT) could restore visual function in RP rat models, showing widespread the subretinal distribution of P3HT nanoparticles and long-term efficacy without triggering retinal inflammation or immune response [73]. Further supporting its potential, Francia and co-workers demonstrated that P3HT nanoparticles restored cortical visual responses in advanced-stage RP rats, even after photoreceptor degeneration [74]. Collectively, these findings indicate the biocompatibility and short-term therapeutic efficacy of non-traditional delivery systems.

6.2. Combination Therapies

Combining gene therapy with other treatment modalities, such as stem cell therapy and retinal implants, represents a promising future direction for enhancing therapeutic outcomes in RP. By integrating these approaches, researchers aim to simultaneously target both genetic defects and cellular degeneration. Several studies have explored the feasibility and efficacy of these combination therapies. MacLaren et al. emphasized that gene and cell-based therapies should be viewed as complementary strategies, with gene therapy offering the greatest benefit in early stages where viable photoreceptors are still present, and stem cell transplantation being more applicable in the advanced stages marked by widespread retinal cell degeneration [13].

Furthermore, Sahel and co-workers provided compelling clinical evidence supporting the integration of optogenetic therapy and retinal prosthetics in a first reported case; by delivering optogenetic gene constructs intravitreally and combining this intervention with light-stimulating goggles, they achieved the partial restoration of visual function in a blind RP patient, underscoring the potential of combined genetic-device interventions [46]. Collectively, these findings emphasize the substantial potential of multimodal therapeutic strategies to address the complex pathology of RP and enhance patient outcomes.

6.3. Regulatory and Ethical Issues

As therapeutic strategies for RP rapidly advance, navigating regulatory pathways and addressing ethical considerations will be critical to translating novel gene therapies into clinical practice. Gene therapies, including advanced vectors and combinational approaches, must undergo rigorous assessment by regulatory authorities such as the U.S. Food and Drug Administration (FDA) and the European Medicines Agency (EMA). The regulatory approval process involves multiple phases of clinical trials designed to thoroughly evaluate safety, efficacy, and long-term outcomes, often requiring extensive follow-up data to substantiate therapeutic benefits and identify potential risks [75]. The landmark approval of Luxturna® (voretigene neparvovec-rzyl), an AAV-based gene therapy for inherited retinal dystrophy caused by *RPE65* mutations, exemplifies the complexity and rigor of these processes and has paved the way for future RP therapies [28].

In parallel with regulatory challenges, ethical concerns surrounding gene therapies for RP must also be carefully considered. Genetic manipulation, particularly techniques involving gene editing or germline modifications, raises significant ethical questions related to potential off-target effects, long-term safety, and the implications of irreversible genomic alterations [76]. Moreover, equitable access to emerging gene therapies remains a significant concern due to their typically high costs, potentially limiting availability to select populations and exacerbating existing healthcare disparities [77]. Ensuring fair distribution and access to these therapies will necessitate ongoing dialogue between researchers, clinicians, policymakers, and patient advocacy groups.

As treatments for patients with RP evolve toward personalized, multimodal interventions, addressing these regulatory and ethical challenges will be crucial to ensuring safe, effective, and accessible therapies for patients worldwide.

6.4. The Path Forward for RP Patients

Advancements in the molecular understanding of RP, along with significant progress in gene therapy platforms, are guiding the way for more personalized treatment strategies for patients with diverse genetic subtypes. Due to RP caused by mutations in over 80 different genes, its genetic heterogeneity poses a major therapeutic challenge. However, recent studies emphasize that expanding genetic screening and variant classification may facilitate the development of mutation-specific therapies [78].

Promising advancements are emerging for specific subtypes such as *RPE65-*, *RPGR-*, and *USH2A*-associated RP. These targeted gene therapy approaches are currently under investigation in clinical trials, with the potential to advance towards further stages of development. Furthermore, innovative non-viral delivery systems, nucleic acid base editing, and CRISPR/Cas9 gene-editing technologies are being explored to expand the spectrum of treatable mutations and address the limitations associated with vector capacity and delivery efficiency [12,78]. These advancements, in addition to the increasing efforts in clinical trial development, suggest that gene therapy may soon evolve from experimental intervention to a standard therapeutic modality for specific genetic subsets of RP.

7. Conclusions

Genetic therapy has reshaped the treatment landscape of RP, shifting from symptomatic management toward targeted molecular interventions. Advances in gene replacement (e.g., Luxturna® for *RPE65*), gene editing (e.g., EDIT-101 for *CEP290*), RNA-based modulation, and optogenetic therapy have demonstrated clinical and preclinical success across various RP genotypes. Additionally, novel delivery strategies, including engineered AAV serotypes and nanoparticle platforms, are helping overcome packaging and transduction limitations, expanding the range of targetable mutations, including those previously considered untreatable due to gene size.

Despite these successes, the therapeutic potential of genetic interventions in RP will depend on overcoming several key challenges, including improving delivery efficiency, addressing immune responses, and ensuring long-term safety and efficacy. Given RP's considerable genetic and phenotypic heterogeneity, precision medicine guided by early genetic diagnosis is essential to identify patients to mutation-specific therapies and implement personalized treatment strategies.

Looking ahead, the translation of experimental therapies into standard clinical practice will require rigorous long-term safety monitoring, scalable delivery systems, and equitable access frameworks. Ultimately, these innovative approaches offer hope to transform the prognosis of patients with RP from progressive vision loss to a future where disease stabilization, and even functional recovery, becomes a realistic goal.

Author Contributions: Conceptualization, R.A.M.C. and N.I.; methodology, R.A.M.C. and N.I.; resources, N.I. and A.E.; data curation, R.A.M.C.; writing—original draft preparation, R.A.M.C.; writing—review and editing, R.A.M.C., N.I. and A.E.; visualization, R.A.M.C.; supervision, N.I. and A.E.; project administration, R.A.M.C., N.I. and A.E.; funding acquisition, none. All authors have read and agreed to the published version of the manuscript.

Funding: This research received no external funding.

Data Availability Statement: No new data were created or analyzed during this study. Data sharing is not applicable to this article.

Conflicts of Interest: A. Emanuelli is owner of Emanuelli Research and Development, Retina Care, where most of the treatments proposed in the review are offered to RP patients.

Abbreviations

The following abbreviations are used in this manuscript:

AAV	Adeno-Associated Virus
AI	Artificial Intelligence
AON	Antisense Oligonucleotide
BCVA	Best-Corrected Visual Acuity
CEP290	Centrosomal Protein of 290 kDa
CRISPR	Clustered Regularly Interspaced Short Palindromic Repeats
ERGs	Electroretinograms
FST	Full-Field Light Sensitivity Threshold
ILM	Inner Limiting Membrane
IRDs	Inherited Retinal Diseases
LCA	Leber Congenital Amaurosis
MLMT	Multi-Luminance Mobility Test
MSNs	Mesoporous Silica Nanoparticles
ONL	Outer Nuclear Layer
P3HT	Poly(3-Hexylthiophene)
PRPF31	Pre-mRNA Processing Factor 31
RHO	Rhodopsin
RP	Retinitis Pigmentosa
RPGR	Retinitis Pigmentosa GTPase Regulator
RPE	Retinal Pigment Epithelium
siRNA	Small Interfering RNA
shRNA	Short Hairpin RNA
UPR	Unfolded Protein Response
USH2A	Usher Syndrome Type 2A

References

1. Verbakel, S.K.; van Huet, R.A.C.; Boon, C.J.F.; den Hollander, A.I.; Collin, R.W.J.; Klaver, C.C.W.; Hoyng, C.B.; Roepman, R.; Klevering, B.J. Non-syndromic retinitis pigmentosa. *Prog. Retin. Eye Res.* **2018**, *66*, 157–186. [CrossRef] [PubMed]
2. Boughman, J.A.; Conneally, P.M.; Nance, W.E. Population Genetic Studies of Retinitis Pigmentosa. *Am. J. Hum. Genet.* **1980**, *32*, 223–235. [PubMed]
3. Hartong, D.T.; Berson, E.L.; Dryja, T.P. Retinitis Pigmentosa Prevalence and Inheritance Patterns. 2006; Volume 368. Available online: www.ncbi.nlm.nih.gov/ (accessed on 3 February 2025).
4. Birtel, J.; Gliem, M.; Mangold, E.; Müller, P.L.; Holz, F.G.; Neuhaus, C.; Lenzner, S.; Zahnleiter, D.; Betz, C.; Eisenberger, T.; et al. Next-generation sequencing identifies unexpected genotype-phenotype correlations in patients with retinitis pigmentosa. *PLoS ONE* **2018**, *13*, e0207958. [CrossRef] [PubMed]
5. Daiger, S.P.; Bowne, S.J.; Sullivan, L.S. Perspective on Genes and Mutations Causing Retinitis Pigmentosa. *Arch. Ophthalmol.* **2007**, *125*, 151–158. [CrossRef]
6. Sandberg, M.A.; Rosner, B.; Weigel-DiFranco, C.; McGee, T.L.; Dryja, T.P.; Berson, E.L. Disease course in patients with autosomal recessive retinitis pigmentosa due to the *USH2A* Gene. *Investig. Opthalmol. Vis. Sci.* **2008**, *49*, 5532–5539. [CrossRef]
7. Zhang, Z.; Dai, H.; Wang, L.; Tao, T.; Xu, J.; Sun, X.; Yang, L.; Li, G. Novel mutations of RPGR in Chinese families with X-linked retinitis pigmentosa. *BMC Ophthalmol.* **2019**, *19*, 1–7. [CrossRef]
8. Liu, W.; Liu, S.; Li, P.; Yao, K. Retinitis Pigmentosa: Progress in Molecular Pathology and Biotherapeutical Strategies. *Int. J. Mol. Sci.* **2022**, *23*, 4883. [CrossRef]
9. Berson, E.L.; Rosner, B.; Sandberg, M.A.; Hayes, K.C.; Nicholson, B.W.; Weigel-DiFranco, C.; Willett, W. A Randomized Trial of Vitamin A and Vitamin E Supplementation for Retinitis Pigmentosa. *Arch. Ophthalmol.* **1993**, *111*, 761–772. [CrossRef]
10. de Castro, C.T.M.; Berezovsky, A.; de Castro, D.D.M.; Salomão, S.R. Visual Rehabilitation in Patients with Retinitis Pigmentosa. *Arq. Bras. Oftalmol.* **2006**, *69*, 687–690. (In Portuguese)
11. Colombo, L.; Baldesi, J.; Martella, S.; Quisisana, C.; Antico, A.; Mapelli, L.; Montagner, S.; Primon, A.; Rossetti, L. Managing Retinitis Pigmentosa: A Literature Review of Current Non-Surgical Approaches. *J. Clin. Med.* **2025**, *14*, 330. [CrossRef]
12. Dias, M.F.; Joo, K.; Kemp, J.A.; Fialho, S.L.; Cunha, A.d.S.; Woo, S.J.; Kwon, Y.J. Molecular genetics and emerging therapies for retinitis pigmentosa: Basic research and clinical perspectives. *Prog. Retin. Eye Res.* **2018**, *63*, 107–131. [CrossRef] [PubMed]
13. MacLaren, R.E.; Bennett, J.; Schwartz, S.D. Gene Therapy and Stem Cell Transplantation in Retinal Disease: The New Frontier. *Ophthalmology* **2016**, *123*, S98–S106. [CrossRef] [PubMed]
14. Sorrentino, F.S.; E Gallenga, C.; Bonifazzi, C.; Perri, P. A challenge to the striking genotypic heterogeneity of retinitis pigmentosa: A better understanding of the pathophysiology using the newest genetic strategies. *Eye* **2016**, *30*, 1542–1548. [CrossRef] [PubMed]
15. Moiseyev, G.; Chen, Y.; Takahashi, Y.; Wu, B.X.; Ma, J.-X. RPE65 is the isomerohydrolase in the retinoid visual cycle. *Proc. Natl. Acad. Sci.* **2005**, *102*, 12413–12418. [CrossRef]
16. Huang, W.C.; Wright, A.F.; Roman, A.J.; Cideciyan, A.V.; Manson, F.D.; Gewaily, D.Y.; Schwartz, S.B.; Sadigh, S.; Limberis, M.P.; Bell, P.; et al. *RPGR*-associated retinal degeneration in human X-linked RP and a murine model. *Investig. Opthalmol. Vis. Sci.* **2012**, *53*, 5594–5608. [CrossRef]
17. Tebbe, L.; Mwoyosvi, M.L.; Crane, R.; Makia, M.S.; Kakakhel, M.; Cosgrove, D.; Al-Ubaidi, M.R.; Naash, M.I. The usherin mutation c.2299delG leads to its mislocalization and disrupts interactions with whirlin and VLGR1. *Nat. Commun.* **2023**, *14*, 972. [CrossRef]
18. Athanasiou, D.; Aguila, M.; Bellingham, J.; Li, W.; McCulley, C.; Reeves, P.J.; Cheetham, M.E. The molecular and cellular basis of rhodopsin retinitis pigmentosa reveals potential strategies for therapy. *Prog. Retin. Eye Res.* **2018**, *62*, 1–23. [CrossRef]
19. Olivares-González, L.; Velasco, S.; Campillo, I.; Millán, J.M.; Rodrigo, R. Redox Status in Retinitis Pigmentosa. In *Advances in Experimental Medicine and Biology*; Springer: Berlin/Heidelberg, Germany, 2023; Volume 1415, pp. 443–448. [CrossRef]
20. Campochiaro, P.A.; Mir, T.A. The mechanism of cone cell death in Retinitis Pigmentosa. *Prog. Retin. Eye Res.* **2018**, *62*, 24–37. [CrossRef]
21. Kanan, Y.; Hackett, S.F.; Hsueh, H.T.; Khan, M.; Ensign, L.M.; Campochiaro, P.A. Reduced Inspired Oxygen Decreases Retinal Superoxide Radicals and Promotes Cone Function and Survival in a Model of Retinitis Pigmentosa. *Free. Radic. Biol. Med.* **2023**, *198*, 118–122. [CrossRef]
22. Zabel, M.K.; Zhao, L.; Zhang, Y.; Gonzalez, S.R.; Ma, W.; Wang, X.; Fariss, R.N.; Wong, W.T. Microglial phagocytosis and activation underlying photoreceptor degeneration is regulated by CX3CL1-CX3CR1 signaling in a mouse model of retinitis pigmentosa. *Glia* **2016**, *64*, 1479–1491. [CrossRef]
23. Di Iorio, V.; Karali, M.; Melillo, P.; Testa, F.; Brunetti-Pierri, R.; Musacchia, F.; Condroyer, C.; Neidhardt, J.; Audo, I.; Zeitz, C.; et al. Spectrum of disease severity in patients with X-linked retinitis pigmentosa due to *RPGR* mutations. *Investig. Opthalmol. Vis. Sci.* **2020**, *61*, 36. [CrossRef] [PubMed]

24. Fahim, A.T.; Bowne, S.J.; Sullivan, L.S.; Webb, K.D.; Williams, J.T.; Wheaton, D.K.; Birch, D.G.; Daiger, S.P.; Janecke, A.R. Allelic heterogeneity and genetic modifier loci contribute to clinical variation in males with X-linked retinitis pigmentosa due to rpgr mutations. *PLoS ONE* **2011**, *6*, e23021. [CrossRef] [PubMed]
25. Dvoriantchikova, G.; Lypka, K.R.; Ivanov, D. The Potential Role of Epigenetic Mechanisms in the Development of Retinitis Pigmentosa and Related Photoreceptor Dystrophies. *Front. Genet.* **2022**, *13*, 827274. [CrossRef] [PubMed]
26. Kutsyr, O.; Sánchez-Sáez, X.; Martínez-Gil, N.; de Juan, E.; Lax, P.; Maneu, V.; Cuenca, N. Gradual increase in environmental light intensity induces oxidative stress and inflammation and accelerates retinal neurodegeneration. *Investig. Opthalmol. Vis. Sci.* **2020**, *61*, 1. [CrossRef]
27. Wang, J.-H.; Zhan, W.; Gallagher, T.L.; Gao, G. Recombinant adeno-associated virus as a delivery platform for ocular gene therapy: A comprehensive review. *Mol. Ther.* **2024**, *32*, 4185–4207. [CrossRef]
28. Russell, S.; Bennett, J.; A Wellman, J.; Chung, D.C.; Yu, Z.-F.; Tillman, A.; Wittes, J.; Pappas, J.; Elci, O.; McCague, S.; et al. Efficacy and safety of voretigene neparvovec (AAV2-hRPE65v2) in patients with RPE65 -mediated inherited retinal dystrophy: A randomised, controlled, open-label, phase 3 trial. *Lancet* **2017**, *390*, 849–860. [CrossRef]
29. Cehajic-Kapetanovic, J.; Xue, K.; de la Camara, C.M.-F.; Nanda, A.; Davies, A.; Wood, L.J.; Salvetti, A.P.; Fischer, M.D.; Aylward, J.W.; Barnard, A.R.; et al. Initial results from a first-in-human gene therapy trial on X-linked retinitis pigmentosa caused by mutations in RPGR. *Nat. Med.* **2020**, *26*, 354–359. [CrossRef]
30. Drag, S.; Dotiwala, F.; Upadhyay, A.K. Gene Therapy for Retinal Degenerative Diseases: Progress, Challenges, and Future Directions. *Investig. Opthalmol. Vis. Sci.* **2023**, *64*, 39. [CrossRef]
31. Bucher, K.; Rodríguez-Bocanegra, E.; Dauletbekov, D.; Fischer, M.D. Immune responses to retinal gene therapy using adeno-associated viral vectors–Implications for treatment success and safety. *Prog. Retin. Eye Res.* **2021**, *83*, 100915. [CrossRef]
32. Datta, P.; Rhee, K.-D.; Staudt, R.J.; Thompson, J.M.; Hsu, Y.; Hassan, S.; Drack, A.V.; Seo, S. Delivering large genes using adeno-associated virus and the CRE-lox DNA recombination system. *Hum. Mol. Genet.* **2024**, *33*, 2094–2110. [CrossRef]
33. Tornabene, P.; Trapani, I. Can Adeno-Associated Viral Vectors Deliver Effectively Large Genes? *Hum. Gene Ther.* **2020**, *31*, 47–56. [CrossRef] [PubMed]
34. Ahmad, I. CRISPR/Cas9—A Promising Therapeutic Tool to Cure Blindness: Current Scenario and Future Prospects. *Int. J. Mol. Sci.* **2022**, *23*, 11482. [CrossRef] [PubMed]
35. Wang, H.; La Russa, M.; Qi, L.S. CRISPR/Cas9 in Genome Editing and beyond. *Annu. Rev. Biochem.* **2016**, *85*, 227–264. [CrossRef] [PubMed]
36. Pierce, E.A.; Aleman, T.S.; Jayasundera, K.T.; Ashimatey, B.S.; Kim, K.; Rashid, A.; Jaskolka, M.C.; Myers, R.L.; Lam, B.L.; Bailey, S.T.; et al. Gene Editing for *CEP290* -Associated Retinal Degeneration. *N. Engl. J. Med.* **2024**, *390*, 1972–1984. [CrossRef]
37. Hu, S.; Du, J.; Chen, N.; Jia, R.; Zhang, J.; Liu, X.; Yang, L. In vivo CRISPR/Cas9-mediated genome editing mitigates photoreceptor degeneration in a mouse model of X-linked retinitis pigmentosa. *Investig. Opthalmol. Vis. Sci.* **2020**, *61*, 31. [CrossRef]
38. Brokowski, C.; Adli, M. CRISPR Ethics: Moral Considerations for Applications of a Powerful Tool. *J. Mol. Biol.* **2019**, *431*, 88–101. [CrossRef]
39. Xue, K.; MacLaren, R.E. Antisense oligonucleotide therapeutics in clinical trials for the treatment of inherited retinal diseases. *Expert Opin. Investig. Drugs* **2020**, *29*, 1163–1170. [CrossRef]
40. Grainok, J.; Pitout, I.L.; Chen, F.K.; McLenachan, S.; Jeffery, R.C.H.; Mitrpant, C.; Fletcher, S. A Precision Therapy Approach for Retinitis Pigmentosa 11 Using Splice-Switching Antisense Oligonucleotides to Restore the Open Reading Frame of PRPF31. *Int. J. Mol. Sci.* **2024**, *25*, 3391. [CrossRef]
41. Slijkerman, R.W.; Vaché, C.; Dona, M.; García-García, G.; Claustres, M.; Hetterschijt, L.; A Peters, T.; Hartel, B.P.; Pennings, R.J.; Millan, J.M.; et al. Antisense Oligonucleotide-based Splice Correction for USH2A-associated Retinal Degeneration Caused by a Frequent Deep-intronic Mutation. *Mol. Ther. Nucleic Acids* **2016**, *5*, e381. [CrossRef]
42. Guzman-Aranguez, A.; Loma, P.; Pintor, J. Small-interfering RNAs (siRNAs) as a promising tool for ocular therapy. *Br. J. Pharmacol.* **2013**, *170*, 730–747. [CrossRef]
43. O'rEilly, M.; Palfi, A.; Chadderton, N.; Millington-Ward, S.; Ader, M.; Cronin, T.; Tuohy, T.; Auricchio, A.; Hildinger, M.; Tivnan, A.; et al. RNA Interference–mediated suppression and replacement of human rhodopsin in vivo. *Am. J. Hum. Genet.* **2007**, *81*, 127–135. [CrossRef] [PubMed]
44. Lindner, M.; Gilhooley, M.J.; Hughes, S.; Hankins, M.W. Optogenetics for visual restoration: From proof of principle to translational challenges. *Prog. Retin. Eye Res.* **2022**, *91*, 101089. [CrossRef] [PubMed]
45. De Silva, S.R.; Moore, A.T.; De Silva, S.R.; Moore, A.T. Physiology 2021 symposium 'Photoreceptors in Health and Monogenic Disease. *J. Physiol.* **2022**, *600*, 4623–4632. [CrossRef] [PubMed]
46. Sahel, J.-A.; Boulanger-Scemama, E.; Pagot, C.; Arleo, A.; Galluppi, F.; Martel, J.N.; Degli Esposti, S.; Delaux, A.; de Saint Aubert, J.-B.; de Montleau, C.; et al. Partial recovery of visual function in a blind patient after optogenetic therapy. *Nat. Med.* **2021**, *27*, 1223–1229. [CrossRef]

47. Batabyal, S.; Kim, S.; Carlson, M.; Narcisse, D.; Tchedre, K.; Dibas, A.; Sharif, N.A.; Mohanty, S. Multi-Characteristic Opsin Therapy to Functionalize Retina, Attenuate Retinal Degeneration, and Restore Vision in Mouse Models of Retinitis Pigmentosa. *Transl. Vis. Sci. Technol.* **2024**, *13*, 25. [CrossRef]
48. Toms, M.; Toualbi, L.; Almeida, P.V.; Harbottle, R.; Moosajee, M. Successful large gene augmentation of USH2A with non-viral episomal vectors. *Mol. Ther.* **2023**, *31*, 2755–2766. [CrossRef]
49. Trapani, I.; Colella, P.; Sommella, A.; Iodice, C.; Cesi, G.; de Simone, S.; Marrocco, E.; Rossi, S.; Giunti, M.; Palfi, A.; et al. Effective delivery of large genes to the retina by dual AAV vectors. *EMBO Mol. Med.* **2013**, *6*, 194–211. [CrossRef]
50. Dalkara, D.; Kolstad, K.D.; Caporale, N.; Visel, M.; Klimczak, R.R.; Schaffer, D.V.; Flannery, J.G. Inner limiting membrane barriers to AAV-mediated retinal transduction from the vitreous. *Mol. Ther.* **2009**, *17*, 2096–2102. [CrossRef]
51. Gamlin, P.D.; Alexander, J.J.; Boye, S.L.; Witherspoon, C.D.; Boye, S.E. SubILM injection of AAV for gene delivery to the retina. In *Methods in Molecular Biology*; Humana Press Inc.: Totowa, NJ, USA, 2019; Volume 1950, pp. 249–262. [CrossRef]
52. Maguire, A.M.; Russell, S.; Wellman, J.A.; Chung, D.C.; Yu, Z.-F.; Tillman, A.; Wittes, J.; Pappas, J.; Elci, O.; Marshall, K.A.; et al. Efficacy, Safety, and Durability of Voretigene Neparvovec-rzyl in RPE65 Mutation–Associated Inherited Retinal Dystrophy: Results of Phase 1 and 3 Trials. *Ophthalmology* **2019**, *126*, 1273–1285. [CrossRef]
53. Adam, M.P.; Feldman, J.; Mirzaa, G.M. RPE65-Related Leber Congenital Amaurosis/Early-Onset Severe Retinal Dystrophy. In *GeneReviews*; University of Washington: Seattle, WA, USA, 1993.
54. Nguyen, X.-T.; Moekotte, L.; Plomp, A.S.; Bergen, A.A.; van Genderen, M.M.; Boon, C.J.F. Retinitis Pigmentosa: Current Clinical Management and Emerging Therapies. *Int. J. Mol. Sci.* **2023**, *24*, 7481. [CrossRef]
55. Arbabi, A.; Liu, A.; Ameri, H. Gene Therapy for Inherited Retinal Degeneration. *J. Ocul. Pharmacol. Ther.* **2019**, *35*, 79–97. [CrossRef] [PubMed]
56. Fenner, B.J.; Tan, T.-E.; Barathi, A.V.; Tun, S.B.B.; Yeo, S.W.; Tsai, A.S.H.; Lee, S.Y.; Cheung, C.M.G.; Chan, C.M.; Mehta, J.S.; et al. Gene-Based Therapeutics for Inherited Retinal Diseases. *Front. Genet.* **2022**, *12*, 794805. [CrossRef] [PubMed]
57. Ito, N.; Miura, G.; Shiko, Y.; Kawasaki, Y.; Baba, T.; Yamamoto, S.; Nakazawa, M. Progression Rate of Visual Function and Affecting Factors at Different Stages of Retinitis Pigmentosa. *BioMed Res. Int.* **2022**, *2022*, 7204954. [CrossRef] [PubMed]
58. Maguire, A.M.; Bennett, J.; Aleman, E.M.; Leroy, B.P.; Aleman, T.S. Clinical Perspective: Treating RPE65-Associated Retinal Dystrophy. *Mol. Ther.* **2021**, *29*, 442–463. [CrossRef]
59. Michaelides, M.; Besirli, C.G.; Yang, Y.; DE Guimaraes, T.A.; Wong, S.C.; Huckfeldt, R.M.; Comander, J.I.; Sahel, J.-A.; Shah, S.M.; Tee, J.J.; et al. Phase 1/2 AAV5-hRKp.RPGR (Botaretigene Sparoparvovec) Gene Therapy: Safety and Efficacy in RPGR-Associated X-Linked Retinitis Pigmentosa. *Arch. Ophthalmol.* **2024**, *267*, 122–134. [CrossRef]
60. Gumerson, J.D.; Alsufyani, A.; Yu, W.; Lei, J.; Sun, X.; Dong, L.; Wu, Z.; Li, T. Restoration of RPGR expression in vivo using CRISPR/Cas9 gene editing. *Gene Ther.* **2021**, *29*, 81–93. [CrossRef]
61. Esteban-Medina, M.; Loucera, C.; Rian, K.; Velasco, S.; Olivares-González, L.; Rodrigo, R.; Dopazo, J.; Peña-Chilet, M. The mechanistic functional landscape of retinitis pigmentosa: A machine learning-driven approach to therapeutic target discovery. *J. Transl. Med.* **2024**, *22*, 139. [CrossRef]
62. Gomes, B.; Ashley, E.A.; Drazen, J.M.; Kohane, I.S.; Leong, T.-Y. Artificial Intelligence in Molecular Medicine. *N. Engl. J. Med.* **2023**, *388*, 2456–2465. [CrossRef]
63. Fujinami-Yokokawa, Y.; Ninomiya, H.; Liu, X.; Yang, L.; Pontikos, N.; Yoshitake, K.; Iwata, T.; Sato, Y.; Hashimoto, T.; Tsunoda, K.; et al. Prediction of causative genes in inherited retinal disorder from fundus photography and autofluorescence imaging using deep learning techniques. *Br. J. Ophthalmol.* **2021**, *105*, 1272–1279. [CrossRef]
64. Issa, M.; Sukkarieh, G.; Gallardo, M.; Sarbout, I.; Bonnin, S.; Tadayoni, R.; Milea, D. Applications of artificial intelligence to inherited retinal diseases: A systematic review. *Surv. Ophthalmol.* **2024**, *70*, 255–264. [CrossRef]
65. Wu, K.Y.; Mina, M.; Sahyoun, J.-Y.; Kalevar, A.; Tran, S.D. Retinal Prostheses: Engineering and Clinical Perspectives for Vision Restoration. *Sensors* **2023**, *23*, 5782. [CrossRef] [PubMed]
66. Ho, A.C.; Humayun, M.S.; Dorn, J.D.; da Cruz, L.; Dagnelie, G.; Handa, J.; Barale, P.-O.; Sahel, J.-A.; Stanga, P.E.; Hafezi, F.; et al. Long-Term Results from an Epiretinal Prosthesis to Restore Sight to the Blind. *Ophthalmology* **2015**, *122*, 1547–1554. [CrossRef] [PubMed]
67. Wang, Y.; Tang, Z.; Gu, P. Stem/progenitor cell-based transplantation for retinal degeneration: A review of clinical trials. *Cell Death Dis.* **2020**, *11*, 793. [CrossRef] [PubMed]
68. Chen, X.; Xu, N.; Li, J.; Zhao, M.; Huang, L. Stem cell therapy for inherited retinal diseases: A systematic review and meta-analysis. *Stem Cell Res. Ther.* **2023**, *14*, 286. [CrossRef]
69. Liu, Y.; Chen, S.J.; Li, S.Y.; Qu, L.H.; Meng, X.H.; Wang, Y.; Xu, H.W.; Liang, Z.Q.; Yin, Z.Q. Long-Term safety of human retinal progenitor cell transplantation in retinitis pigmentosa patients. *Stem Cell Res. Ther.* **2017**, *8*, 209. [CrossRef]
70. Pavlou, M.; Schön, C.; Occelli, L.M.; Rossi, A.; Meumann, N.; Boyd, R.F.; Bartoe, J.T.; Siedlecki, J.; Gerhardt, M.J.; Babutzka, S.; et al. Novel AAV capsids for intravitreal gene therapy of photoreceptor disorders. *EMBO Mol. Med.* **2021**, *13*, e13392. [CrossRef]

71. He, X.; Fu, Y.; Xu, Y.; Ma, L.; Chai, P.; Shi, H.; Yao, Y.; Ge, S.; Jia, R.; Wen, X.; et al. A Penetrable AAV2 Capsid Variant for Efficient Intravitreal Gene Delivery to the Retina. *Investig. Opthalmol. Vis. Sci.* **2025**, *66*, 6. [CrossRef]
72. Valdés-Sánchez, L.; Borrego-González, S.; Montero-Sánchez, A.; Massalini, S.; de la Cerda, B.; Díaz-Cuenca, A.; Díaz-Corrales, F.J. Mesoporous Silica-Based Nanoparticles as Non-Viral Gene Delivery Platform for Treating Retinitis Pigmentosa. *J. Clin. Med.* **2022**, *11*, 2170. [CrossRef]
73. Maya-Vetencourt, J.F.; Manfredi, G.; Mete, M.; Colombo, E.; Bramini, M.; Di Marco, S.; Shmal, D.; Mantero, G.; Dipalo, M.; Rocchi, A.; et al. Subretinally injected semiconducting polymer nanoparticles rescue vision in a rat model of retinal dystrophy. *Nat. Nanotechnol.* **2020**, *15*, 698–708. [CrossRef]
74. Francia, S.; Shmal, D.; Di Marco, S.; Chiaravalli, G.; Maya-Vetencourt, J.F.; Mantero, G.; Michetti, C.; Cupini, S.; Manfredi, G.; DiFrancesco, M.L.; et al. Light-induced charge generation in polymeric nanoparticles restores vision in advanced-stage retinitis pigmentosa rats. *Nat. Commun.* **2022**, *13*, 3677. [CrossRef]
75. High, K.A.; Roncarolo, M.G. Gene Therapy. *N. Engl. J. Med.* **2019**, *381*, 455–464. [CrossRef] [PubMed]
76. Ormond, K.E.; Mortlock, D.P.; Scholes, D.T.; Bombard, Y.; Brody, L.C.; Faucett, W.A.; Garrison, N.A.; Hercher, L.; Isasi, R.; Middleton, A.; et al. Human Germline Genome Editing. *Am. J. Hum. Genet.* **2017**, *101*, 167–176. [CrossRef] [PubMed]
77. Malvasi, M.; Casillo, L.; Avogaro, F.; Abbouda, A.; Vingolo, E.M. Gene Therapy in Hereditary Retinal Dystrophies: The Usefulness of Diagnostic Tools in Candidate Patient Selections. *Int. J. Mol. Sci.* **2023**, *24*, 13756. [CrossRef] [PubMed]
78. Liu, Y.; Zong, X.; Cao, W.; Zhang, W.; Zhang, N.; Yang, N. Gene Therapy for Retinitis Pigmentosa: Current Challenges and New Progress. *Biomolecules* **2024**, *14*, 903. [CrossRef]

medicina

MDPI

Article

Comparison of Adhesion of Immortalized Human Iris-Derived Cells and Fibronectin on Phakic Intraocular Lenses Made of Different Polymer Base Materials

Kei Ichikawa [1,2], Yoshiki Tanaka [1], Rie Horai [1], Yu Kato [3], Kazuo Ichikawa [1,*] and Naoki Yamamoto [3,4]

[1] Chukyo Eye Clinic, Nagoya 456-0032, Aichi, Japan; kei@chukyogroup.jp (K.I.); ytanaka@chukyomedical.co.jp (Y.T.); horai@chukyomedical.co.jp (R.H.)
[2] General Aoyama Hospital, Toyokawa 441-0103, Aichi, Japan
[3] Center for Society-Academia Collaboration, Research Promotion Headquarters, Fujita Health University, Toyoake 470-1192, Aichi, Japan; yu.toki@fujita-hu.ac.jp (Y.K.); naokiy@fujita-hu.ac.jp (N.Y.)
[4] International Center for Cell and Gene Therapy, Research Promotion Headquarters, Fujita Health University, Toyoake 470-1192, Aichi, Japan
* Correspondence: ichikawa@chukyogroup.jp; Tel.: +81-52-884-7976

Abstract: *Background and Objectives:* Posterior chamber phakic implantable contact lenses (Phakic-ICL) are widely used for refractive correction due to their efficacy and safety, including minimal corneal endothelial cell loss. The Collamer-based EVO+ Visian implantable contact lens (ICL), manufactured from Collamer, which is a blend of collagen and hydroxyethyl methacrylate (HEMA), has demonstrated excellent long-term biocompatibility and optical clarity. Recently, hydrophilic acrylic Phakic-ICLs, such as the Implantable Phakic Contact Lens (IPCL), have been introduced. This study investigated the material differences among Phakic-ICLs and their interaction with fibronectin (FN), which has been reported to adhere to intraocular lens (IOL) surfaces following implantation. The aim was to compare Collamer, IPCL, and LENTIS lenses (used as control) in terms of FN distribution and cell adhesion using a small number of explanted Phakic-ICLs. *Materials and Methods:* Three lens types were analyzed: a Collamer Phakic-ICL (EVO+ Visian ICL), a hydrophilic acrylic IPCL, and a hydrophilic acrylic phakic-IOL (LENTIS). FN distribution and cell adhesion were evaluated across different regions of each lens. An in vitro FN-coating experiment was conducted to assess its effect on cell adhesion. *Results*: All lenses demonstrated minimal FN deposition and cellular adhesion in the central optical zone. A thin FN film was observed on the haptics of Collamer lenses, while FN adhesion was weaker or absent on IPCL and LENTIS surfaces. Following FN coating, Collamer lenses supported more uniform FN film formation; however, this did not significantly enhance cell adhesion. *Conclusions*: Collamer, which contains collagen, promotes FN film formation. Although FN film formation was enhanced, the low cell-adhesive properties of HEMA resulted in minimal cell adhesion even with FN presence. This characteristic may contribute to the long-term transparency and biocompatibility observed clinically. In contrast, hydrophilic acrylic materials used in IPCL and LENTIS demonstrated limited FN interaction. These material differences may influence extracellular matrix protein deposition and biocompatibility in clinical settings, warranting further investigation.

Keywords: implantable contact lens (ICL); phakic implantable contact lens (Phakic-ICL); collamer; implantable phakic contact lens (IPCL); LENTIS comfort; fibronectin (FN)

1. Introduction

A phakic implantable contact lens (Phakic-ICL) is a lens inserted into the eye to correct refractive errors while preserving the natural crystalline lens. Phakic-ICL implantation is a reversible surgical procedure that offers a treatment option for patients with high myopia or corneal abnormalities, such as irregular shape or insufficient thickness. If necessary, the Phakic-ICL can be removed or replaced. It is positioned in the posterior chamber (the space between the iris and crystalline lens) on the posterior surface of the iris. Phakic-ICL implantation was developed in the 1980s, predating the first report of LASIK in 1990 [1,2].

The Implantable Phakic Contact Lens (IPCL) consists of a hybrid semi-hydrophilic acrylic material designed to maintain visual function over extended periods. This material contains high water content and resists the adhesion of foreign substances, such as proteins, to the lens surface [3]. The IPCL has a large optical zone (6.6 mm, diameter) and a trapezoidal aperture rather than a cylindrical one, which helps reduce halos and glare. Seven holes in the optic zone promote aqueous humor circulation, reducing the risk of cataracts and glaucoma. However, since the IPCL material has no affinity for fibronectin (FN), proteins from the aqueous humor may adhere to the lens surface, potentially causing the immune system to recognize it as a foreign body and trigger an immune response. This phenomenon has been observed with other lenses manufactured from hybrid semi-hydrophilic acrylic materials [4].

Two representative Phakic-ICLs are the Implantable Collamer® Lens (Collamer), manufactured by STAAR Surgical, and the IPCL, manufactured by Care Group Sight Solution [5]. The ICL is composed of Collamer, a hydrophilic material made of a copolymer grafted with collagen. This material promotes FN adhesion and enhances hydrophilicity. The lens includes a central port that facilitates gas and nutrient exchange, reducing the risk of cataracts and glaucoma [6]. Collamer consists of a copolymer of hydroxyethyl methacrylate (HEMA) and a UV-absorbing methacrylic monomer (benzophenone), with a small amount of collagen. The material contains 36% water and has <1 ppm of residual monomers in its final hydrated state [7]. Its hydration is uniform throughout the lens. Due to the collagen component, Collamer exhibits affinity for FN, but the limited amount of collagen does not promote broader protein or cell adhesion. Instead, it supports the formation of a monolayer of FN on the lens surface, which inhibits the binding of other aqueous proteins. Because this FN layer is derived from the host, the immune system does not recognize the lens as a foreign body [8–11]. Due to the presence of collagen, studies have reported that FN binds relatively significantly to various cell-extracellular matrix (ECM) interfaces, making it difficult for other ECM proteins to adhere [11].

ECM interactions are complex processes. The ECM not only provides structural support for cells and tissues but also transmits biochemical signals through membrane-spanning receptors that regulate cell proliferation, differentiation, migration, and adhesion. Increased hydrophilicity of a material reduces interfacial energy with water while increasing surface free energy, both of which contribute to reduced cell adhesion. Maximum cell adhesion occurs at a water contact angle of 60° to 70°. Both high hydrophilicity and excessive hydrophobicity can suppress cell adhesion [12]. FN is one of the ECM proteins present in the eye.

Among Phakic-ICLs, posterior chamber lenses are selected for their efficacy and safety, including minimal corneal endothelial cell loss. Collamer lenses have dominated this market sector due to their established safety profile. However, several companies have recently introduced hydrophilic acrylic ICLs. In this study, we investigated the safety characteristics of these newer lenses, focusing on differences in material composition and design. We compared the two most widely used Phakic-ICL, Collamer ICL, and IPCL, regarding their interaction with FN, which forms part of the cellular matrix, including their cellular adhesion properties.

2. Materials and Methods

2.1. Materials

Two types of Phakic-ICL were used in the experiments: Collamer lens (EVO+ VISIAN® Implantable Collamer® Lens VICM5_12.6, STAAR Surgical Co., Lake Forest, CA, USA) with a length of 12.6 mm, an optic diameter of 5.0–6.1 mm, and a power of –7.50 diopters; and IPCL lens (Implantable Phakic Contact Lens V2.0, Care Group Sight Solution LLP, Gujarat, India) with a length of 12.5 mm, an optic diameter of 6.60 mm, and a power of –7.50 diopters. Additionally, one type of Phakic-ICL was included in this study: LENTIS (LENTIS® Comfort Acrylic Foldable Intraocular Lens LS-313 MF15, Santen Pharmaceutical Co., Ltd., Osaka, Japan), with a length of 11.0 mm, an optic diameter of 6.0 mm, and a power of +10.0 diopters. The LENTIS lens, manufactured from hydrophilic acrylic material, served as a control for comparison with the Collamer and IPCL lenses in this study (Supplementary Table S1).

2.2. Explanted Lenses

We analyzed the surface characteristics of explanted lenses from three cases: two involving Collamer lenses and one involving an IPCL (Table 1).

- Case 1: A patient with a Collamer lens implanted 171 months previously.
- Case 2: A patient with a Collamer lens implanted 178 months previously.
- Case 3: A patient with an IPCL implanted 16 months previously.

Table 1. Case information.

Case	Age/Gender	Reasons for Removal	Treatment	Lens Vault (Preoperative)	Post-Operative Uncorrected Visual Acuity
Case 1	39/Female	Due to low vault	lens replacement	52 μm	1.5 (lens vault: 1CT)
Case 2	45/Male	For monovision (OD: 0.9, OS: 0.4)	lens replacement	261 μm	OD: 1.2, OS: 1.5
Case 3	52/Male	hard to see	lens extraction	666 μm	1.2

This retrospective study was approved by the Medical Research Ethics Committee (Chukyo Eye Clinic Ethics Committee, No. 20250519095) and adhered to the tenets of the Declaration of Helsinki. In this study, Phakic-ICLs that were removed and would otherwise be discarded were used as research materials; therefore, there was no invasion or intervention. We obtained consent from patients to use the removed Phakic-ICLs and medical information under the condition that all data would be anonymized to prevent patient identification. Furthermore, following ethics committee review and given that only anonymized patient and medical information were used retrospectively, we disclosed the research content of this study using an opt-out method.

2.3. Immunohistochemical Staining of FN Using Explanted Phakic-ICL

After explantation, each lens was immediately placed in fresh BSS Plus solution (Alcon Japan Ltd., Tokyo, Japan), washed, and temporarily stored. The lenses were then fixed in 4% paraformaldehyde (FUJIFILM Wako Pure Chemical Corp., Osaka, Japan) at room temperature for 15 min, followed by a 15 min wash in phosphate-buffered saline (PBS, FUJIFILM Wako Pure Chemical Corp.) at room temperature. A protein blocking solution (Cat. No. X0909, Agilent Technologies, Inc., Santa Clara, CA, USA) was applied at room temperature for 10 min. Excess blocking solution was aspirated, and rabbit polyclonal anti-fibronectin antibody (Cat. No. ab2413, 1:50 dilution, Abcam plc., Cambridge, UK) was added and incubated overnight at 4 °C. After washing with PBS, the fluorescent secondary antibody, Donkey anti-Rabbit IgG (H + L), Highly Cross-Adsorbed, Alexa Fluor™ 488 (Cat. No. A-21206, 1:500 dilution, Thermo Fisher Scientific Inc., Waltham, MA, USA), was applied and incubated at 37 °C for 2 h. The samples were then washed with PBS, observed, and photographed using a fluorescence inverted microscope (Olympus Power IX71, Olympus Corp., Tokyo, Japan) and a digital camera system (Olympus DP-51, Olympus Corp.).

2.4. Experimental FN Fluorescence Detection

Five micrograms (5 μg) of preliminarily green fluorescently labeled FN (HiLyte Fluor™ 488-labeled, Cytoskeleton, Inc., Denver, CO, USA) was dissolved in 1 mL of BSS, then added to a Falcon® 24-well cell culture plate (Corning Incorporated, Corning, NY, USA), with one well used for each lens. Three types of lenses were tested: lenses precoated with FN (three lenses per type) and lenses in BSS only (one lens per type). The lenses were incubated at 37 °C for 36 h. After incubation, the lenses were thrice washed with BSS before observation. FN fluorescence intensity on the lenses was measured using the real-time imaging microplate reader Spark® Cyto (Tecan Group Ltd., Männedorf, Zürich, Switzerland), and further analyzed using an inverted fluorescence microscope (Olympus Power IX71, Olympus Corp.) and digital camera system (Olympus DP-51, Olympus Corp.). Each lens was tested three times in a single experiment, and the same experiment was repeated twice.

2.5. Cell Adhesion Experiments

The lenses used were Collamer, IPCL, and LENTIS lenses, which were precoated under the same conditions as the FN adhesion experiments (5 μg/mL in BSS) or placed in BSS only. A total of 18 lenses of each type were used.

Immortalized human iris epithelial cells (iHIE-NY2) were used in cell adhesion experiments because phakic ICLs may come into contact with iris epithelial cells. Briefly, a portion of iris tissue removed during partial iridectomy from patients with angle-closure glaucoma was cultured. The culture conditions, gene transfer method, and vector information were as previously reported [13,14]. Cells were seeded by adding 100 μL of cell suspension at a concentration of 1×10^5 cells/mL per lens and allowing them to stand for 2 h before adding 1 mL of culture medium.

Cell growth was observed and recorded using an inverted microscope (Olympus Power IX71, Olympus Corporation, Tokyo, Japan) and a digital camera system (Olympus DP-51, Olympus Corporation). Cell proliferation was measured using Cell Counting Kit-8 (Dojindo Laboratories Co., Ltd., Kumamoto, Japan), containing 2-(2-methoxy-4-nitrophenyl)-3-(4-nitrophenyl)-5-(2,4-disulfophenyl)-2H-tetrazolium monosodium salt (WST-8). Cultures were performed in triplicate for each sample, and cell adhesion and proliferation were evaluated after 1, 5, and 10 days of culture.

Cell counting Kit-8 reagent, diluted 1:10 in culture medium, was added to each well and allowed to react for 3 h at 37.0 °C in a 5% CO_2 incubator. The supernatant from the culture medium was then transferred to a 96-well, clear, TC-treated multiple-well plate (P/N: 3599, Corning Inc.), and the absorbance at 450 nm was measured using a microplate reader (Multiskan FC, Thermo Fisher Scientific Inc., Waltham, MA, USA). Five lenses were used in each experiment, with one lens serving as a negative control for each lens type. The same experiment was repeated three times.

2.6. Statistical Analysis

Data are presented as mean ± standard deviation (SD) and were analyzed using Kruskal–Wallis one-way ANOVA, followed by Scheffé's post hoc test for comparisons among three or more independent groups, using SPSS Statistics 24 (IBM Corporation, New York, NY, USA).

3. Results

The following results describe the FN adhesion status in explanted Collamer, IPCL, and LENTIS lenses, FN adhesion in experimental lenses, and cell adhesion to lenses with and without FN coating.

3.1. FN and Cell Adhesion Status in Explanted Lenses

In both Collamer and IPCL explants, the central optical zone area was almost devoid of FN and cellular components. In contrast, FN and cellular components were observed adhering to the four haptics in Collamer and to portions of the six haptics in IPCL, as well as at the peripheral areas where the lens contacts the iris. In Case 1, slight cellular components adhered to the iris-contact area, and a thin FN film was observed in that region. In Case 2, FN adhered as a thin film, particularly on the haptics. In Case 3, cell aggregates were observed on some haptics, and FN was observed adhering to the haptics, though not uniformly distributed (Figure 1).

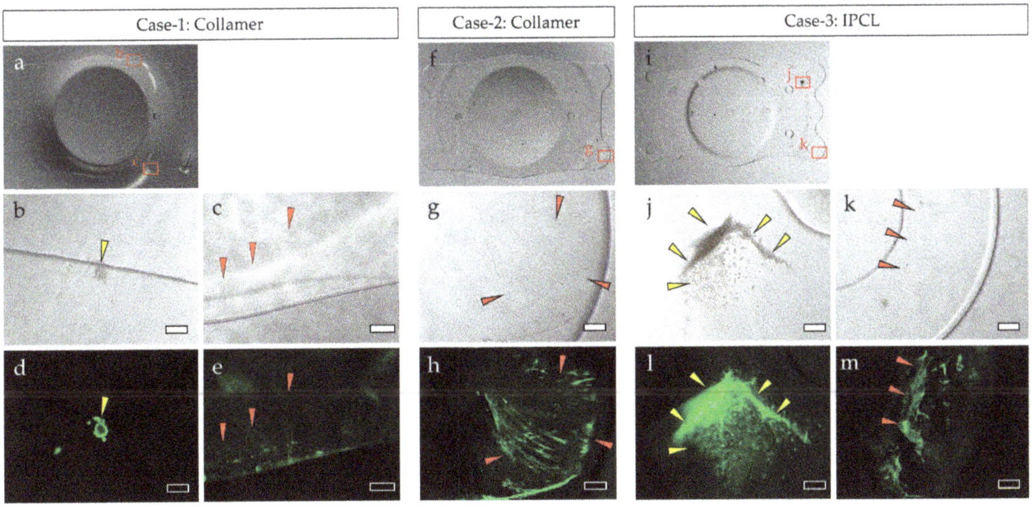

Figure 1. Surface analysis of explanted ICLs: Collamer explanted in Case 1 (**a**–**e**), Collamer explanted in Case 2 (**f**,**g**), and IPCL explanted in Case 3 (**i**–**m**). Macrograph (**a**,**f**,**i**), phase contrast microscope photographs (**b**,**c**,**g**,**j**,**k**), and fluorescent microscope photographs of FN stained with antibody (**d**,**e**,**h**,**l**,**m**). Images show the same locations (**b** and **d**, **c** and **e**, **g** and **h**, **j** and **l**, **k** and **m**). Yellow arrows: cellular components. Red arrows: FN. Bar = 200 μm (**b**,**d**,**g**,**h**,**j**,**k**,**l**,**m**) or bar = 500 μm (**c**,**e**).

3.2. Evaluation of FN Adhesion

After incubation with fluorescently labeled FN solution, FN adhered to the optical edge and center of the Collamer lens optic, as observed using fluorescence microscopy. The Collamer lens demonstrated film-like FN distribution across these regions. In contrast, IPCL and control LENTIS lenses showed increased fluorescence compared to uncoated lenses, but the FN distribution was not uniform or film-like in pattern (Figure 2a). When fluorescently labeled FN was quantified using a real-time imaging microplate reader, Collamer demonstrated the highest fluorescence intensity, significantly greater than that observed in IPCL and LENTIS lenses (Figure 2b).

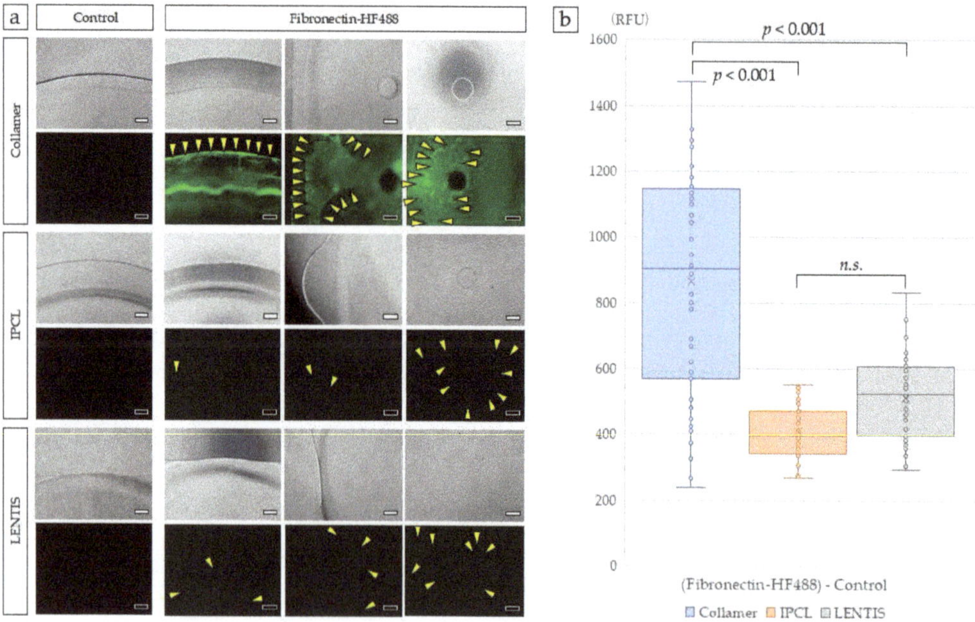

Figure 2. Surface analysis of ICLs incubated with FN. Collamer demonstrated film-like fluorescence at the optic edge, mid-optic region, and optic center. Slight green fluorescence was observed in IPCL and LENTIS compared to controls. Yellow arrowheads indicate FN detected as discrete points (**a**). Each lens was photographed with a 40× objective lens. Fluorescence intensity was quantified using a real-time imaging microplate reader (**b**). Statistical analysis was performed using Kruskal–Wallis one-way ANOVA. Bar = 500 μm. The n.s. was not significant.

3.3. Effect of FN Coating on Cell Adhesion and Proliferation

iHIE-NY2 cells were seeded onto FN-coated and uncoated Collamer, IPCL, and LENTIS lenses and cultured at 37 °C in a 5% CO_2 incubator for 1, 5, and 10 days. Positive controls were established by culturing the same number of cells in standard cell culture wells. Cell adhesion was generally enhanced by FN coating across all three lens types.

On Collamer lenses, cells adhered to the optic center on day 1, but the number of adherent cells decreased by day 10. In contrast, the haptics demonstrated gradual cell proliferation, with marked adhesion observed within the haptic holes. IPCL lenses exhibited fewer adherent cells in both the optic center and haptics compared to Collamer. Minimal cell adhesion was observed within the haptic holes of IPCL. LENTIS lenses also demonstrated minimal adhesion to the optic surface; however, sheet-like clusters of adherent cells were observed in some haptic areas. The number of adherent cells on both IPCL and LENTIS was significantly lower than in positive control wells (Figure 3). The haptic holes of Collamer appeared smaller and had rougher inner surfaces compared to IPCL, which had larger, more rounded holes.

Cell activity, as measured by WST-8, demonstrated a slight overall increase over time across all lens types. On day 1, cell activity was significantly lower in uncoated Collamer, IPCL, and LENTIS lenses compared to the FN-coated LENTIS lens ($p < 0.05$). On day 5, only the uncoated IPCL lens showed significantly lower activity than FN-coated LENTIS lenses ($p < 0.05$). By day 10, no significant differences in cell activity were observed between lens types or coating conditions (Figure 4). Using FN-coated LENTIS as a reference, all lens types demonstrated increased cellular activity over time. Across all lens types, FN-coated lenses consistently exhibited higher activity than their uncoated counterparts (Table 2).

Statistically significant differences were observed in cell adhesion and cell activity based on the presence or absence of FN coating. However, while the FN-coated LENTIS control demonstrated the highest cell adhesion among all experimental groups, the increases in cell adhesion and cell activity across all lens types were only slight, and no visible lens opacification due to cell adhesion was observed.

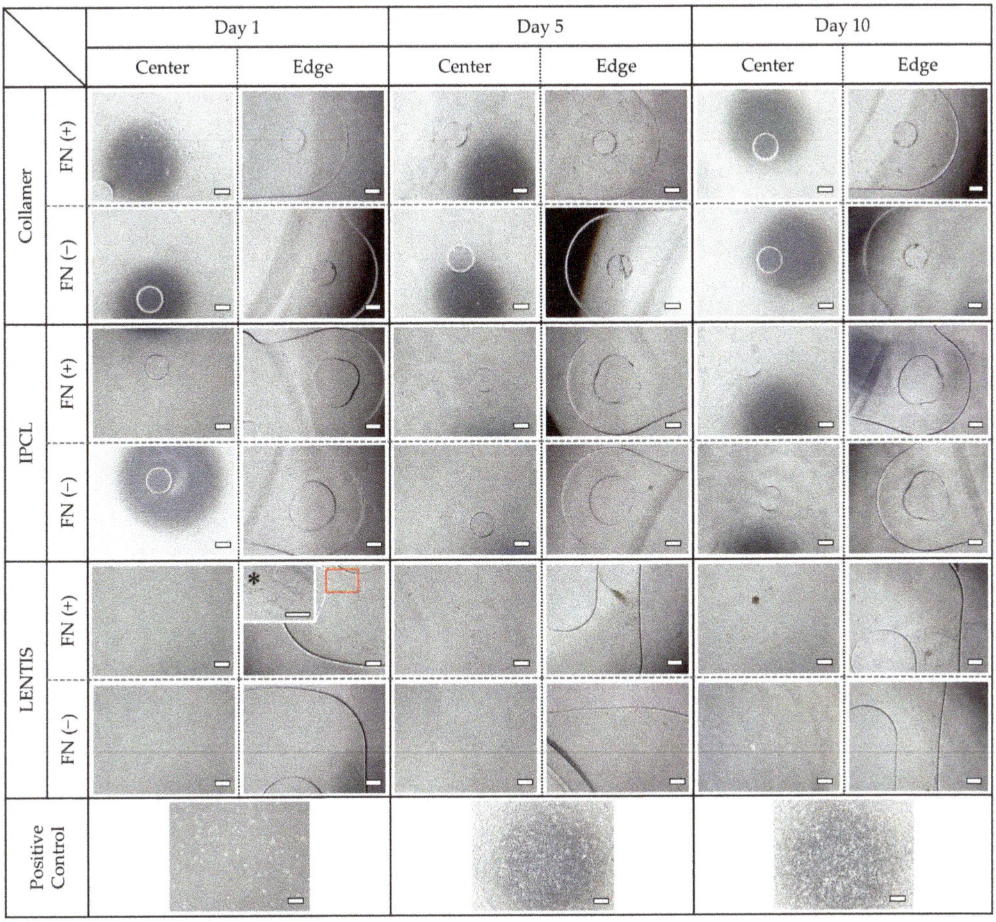

Figure 3. Cell adhesion to each lens with and without FN coating. Phase contrast images of the optic center and haptics on days 1, 5, and 10 of culture. Positive controls were cultured in standard cell culture wells with the same number of seeded cells. All images were taken with a 40× objective lens. * Magnification of the haptics of FN-coated LENTIS was taken with a 100× objective lens. Bar = 500 µm.

Table 2. Comparison of cell activity measured by WST-8, using FN-coated LENTIS lenses as the reference.

Lens	FN Coating	Day 1	Day 5	Day 10
Collamer	Yes	32.1%	75.0%	93.8%
	No	26.8%	39.3%	70.3%
IPCL	Yes	12.5%	60.7%	66.1%
	No	12.5%	23.2%	59.4%
LENTIS	Yes	100%	100%	100%
	No	41.1%	64.3%	67.2%

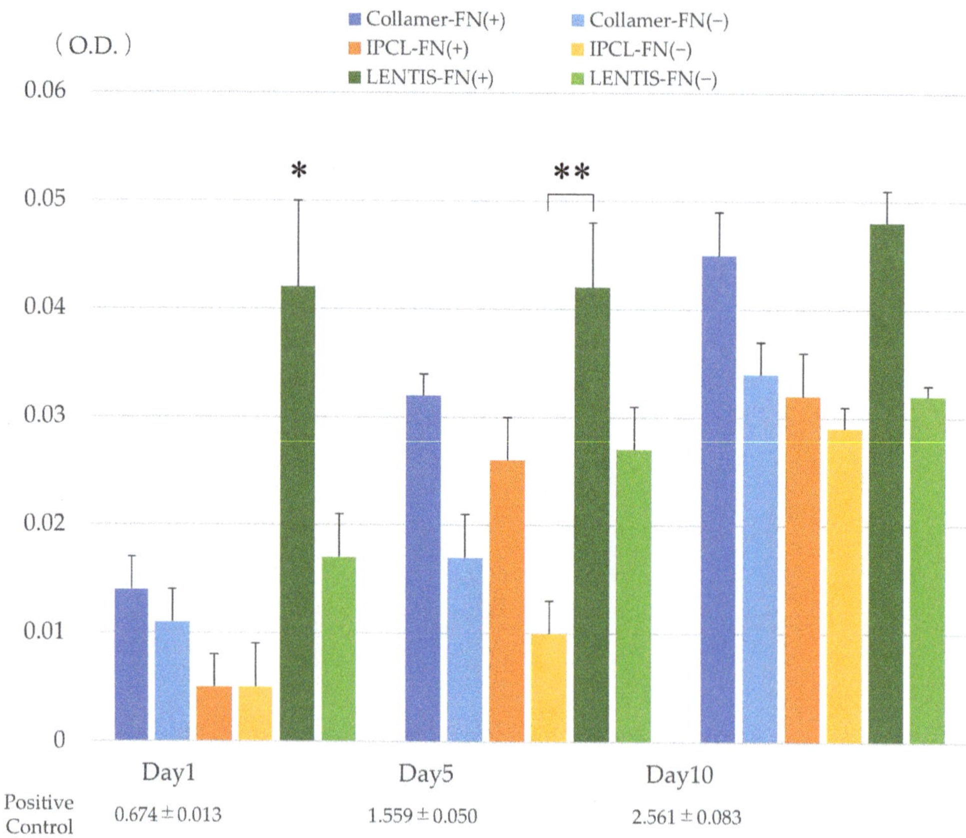

Figure 4. Cellular activity on each lens with or without FN coating measured using WST-8 on days 1, 5, and 10 of incubation. * Significant difference ($p < 0.05$) between FN-coated LENTIS lenses and other lenses on day 1. ** Significantly lower cell activity ($p < 0.05$) in uncoated IPCL lenses compared to FN-coated LENTIS lenses on day 5. The positive control represents cell activity in standard culture wells seeded with the same number of cells. O.D. indicates optical density (absorbance). Statistical analysis was performed using Kruskal–Wallis one-way ANOVA.

4. Discussion

Phakic-ICLs provide superior visual quality, faster recovery, greater refractive accuracy and stability, preservation of accommodation, and reversibility compared to corneal refractive surgeries such as LASIK [9,15,16].

Collamer is a copolymer comprising HEMA and grafted collagen. It has a soft texture due to the unique mechanical properties of its polymer meshwork (Poisson's ratio: 0.4999; elongation at break: 1000%). The presence of collagen imparts a negative surface charge, repelling negatively charged proteins and reducing biofilm formation. Collamer demonstrates excellent biocompatibility and maintains long-term intraocular stability. ICLs manufactured from Collamer received CE marking in Europe in 2003, FDA approval in the U.S. in 2005, and the Ministry of Health, Labour and Welfare approval in Japan in 2010. ICL surgery is now performed in over 70 countries and is recognized alongside LASIK as a standard refractive correction procedure. The Collamer ICL has undergone several design iterations to achieve its current optimized form [6,17,18].

In the early 1990s, Fyodorov of the Moscow Eye Institute introduced the posterior chamber Phakic-ICL. His silicone model, a predecessor of the PRL (Phakic Refractive Lens, Carl Zeiss Meditec), was discontinued due to cataract formation and zonular damage, as the material was too rigid (Poisson's ratio: 0.47) for delicate intraocular tissues. This experience led to the development of the much softer Collamer material at the same institute. Incorporating collagen into Collamer improved its biocompatibility by enabling FN monolayer formation on the lens surface, effectively shielding it from immune recognition [19]. Furthermore, the FN monolayer formed on Collamer may contribute to the rotational stability of the intraocular lens, although further investigation is needed regarding this hypothesis.

Our focus on FN in this study was based on previous research in the ophthalmic field demonstrating that ECM components continuously affect cellular behavior when corneal epithelial cells are cultured on plates coated with laminin, FN, and type IV collagen [20]. Furthermore, the major differences between Collamer and IPCL are their base materials, HEMA versus acrylic, and the presence or absence of collagen. It has been reported that covalently bonding collagen to HEMA-based Phakic-ICLs of similar shape to Collamer results in FN inhibiting the non-specific adsorption of other proteins [10].

The IPCL comprises a hybrid hydrophilic acrylic material with high water content, designed to minimize protein adhesion and maintain long-term visual function. It has a large (6.6 mm) optical zone and a trapezoidal aperture to reduce halos and glare. Seven peripheral holes improve aqueous humor circulation, decreasing the risks of cataract and glaucoma formation [3]. However, compared to Collamer, our study results demonstrated that IPCL materials lack affinity for FN. Consequently, proteins from aqueous humor can adhere to the lens surface, potentially triggering immune recognition and inflammatory responses [8–11].

The ECM provides a structural scaffold for cell adhesion. FN binds to collagen in the ECM, while integrins on cell membranes bind to FN, facilitating cell attachment. However, highly hydrophilic surfaces tend to have lower interfacial energy and higher surface free energy, which weakens cell adhesion. Therefore, hydrophilic lenses such as IPCL may hinder cell attachment [12].

This study focused on the effect of FN in cell adhesion. While FN and bovine serum albumin enhance cell adhesion on various materials, HEMA alone demonstrates minimal adhesion under most conditions [8]. However, in Collamer lenses, FN adheres to the grafted porcine collagen, forming a protective membrane-like layer. In contrast, FN adhered only in discrete patches to IPCL and LENTIS lenses. Since FN adhesion increases on more hydrophilic surfaces (those with lower contact angles), our findings suggest that Collamer's superior FN adhesion reflects its more hydrophilic properties among the lenses studied [21].

Cell adhesion was significantly lower on all lenses compared to positive controls. Within individual lenses, the haptic regions tended to support greater cell adhesion than the optic regions, a trend that was enhanced by FN coating. Additionally, cells adhered to the inner surfaces of the haptic holes in Collamer lenses. These holes are smaller than those in IPCL, and differences in inner surface texture and overall geometry may influence adhesion patterns. Although LENTIS is an IOL rather than a Phakic-ICL, it was included as a material control because it is manufactured from hydrophilic acrylic material similar to IPCL. The haptics of Phakic-ICLs are inserted into the narrow space between the iris and crystalline lens. Since the iris is constantly mobile due to factors such as light exposure, inflammation caused by lens material poses a risk of adhesion to the iris tissue. The explanted Collamer lenses demonstrated membrane-like FN attachment to the haptics without iris adhesion, allowing successful extraction. These results suggest that although FN attachment occurred, cellular adhesion remained minimal, maintaining biocompatibility and allowing sustained transparency over the long term. Furthermore, in 342 eyes examined 3 yrs after Collamer implantation, laser flare photometry and cellular response measurements, which quantify anterior chamber inflammation, showed zero flare values and cellular responses, indicating excellent biocompatibility [11]. Based on our study results, Collamer demonstrated high FN adhesion and attachment properties, but we attribute the lack of increased cell adhesion to the inherent properties of both the collagen component and the HEMA base material. We hypothesize that improved FN biocompatibility may lead to reduced foreign body reactions over the long term, as fewer deposits accumulate on the lens surface, thereby maintaining Collamer transparency. The lack of increased cell adhesion is attributed to the inherent properties of HEMA materials, which are naturally less conducive to cell adhesion.

Surface modification of biomaterials is known to improve blood compatibility [22] and enhance cell adhesion and proliferation [23]. FN, a well-characterized ECM glycoprotein, is abundant in connective tissue and plasma [24] and mediates cell-ECM interactions by binding to ECM components and integrin receptors [25]. Thin FN coatings reduce monocytes and platelet activation, making then suitable for cardiovascular implants [26]. FN coating improves biomaterial biocompatibility by promoting endothelialization via integrin-mediated binding [27]. FN is used in orthopedic and regenerative medicine applications to coat implantable materials [28]. In ophthalmology, FN-coated acrylic IOLs demonstrate improved hydrophilicity [29]. The aqueous humor contains FN at concentrations approximately 100-fold lower than plasma [30], which allows FN to remain as a stable monolayer. The FN layer naturally forming on Collamer enhances ICL biocompatibility. Anterior flare and inflammatory cell measurements obtained up to 3 yrs after Collamer insertion (293 cases, 525 eyes) showed no anterior flare or cellular reaction in >99.6% of cases [11].

Chemical surface modification of HEMA to covalently bind collagen has been shown to promote selective FN binding, mimicking the ECM microenvironment and suppressing macrophage activation while reducing non-specific protein adsorption [10]. FN's safety and efficacy have been validated in both in vitro cell proliferation assays and in vivo transplantation studies [10].

This study has several limitations. First, we focused exclusively on FN among ECM proteins. Since FN exists in multiple isoforms, a more detailed investigation is warranted. Second, aqueous humor contains various other ECM proteins (such as laminin and type IV collagen), necessitating the analysis of all substances adhering to implanted lens surfaces. Third, the culture period was limited to 10 days, assuming it is unlikely that significant changes in adhesion or proliferation would occur beyond this timeframe, but this is unconfirmed. The use of only iris-derived cells limits generalizability, as responses of fibroblasts or immune cells were not evaluated. Furthermore, the small number of explanted cases (3 cases) from a limited patient population restricts the generalizability of findings to diverse patient populations with varying medical conditions, plus the small sample size prevented systematic analysis of the influence of implantation duration (16 vs. 171–178 months), which may be a confounding variable.

5. Conclusions

FN formed a membrane-like layer on the surface of Collamer, likely due to its collagen component and biological compatibility. Experimental data demonstrated greater FN adhesion to Collamer compared to IPCL, supporting the role of collagen in facilitating ECM membrane formation. Although Collamer demonstrated enhanced FN adhesion, this did not result in increased cell adhesion, presumably because HEMA-based materials have low cell-adhesive properties. However, the enhanced adhesion of FN suggests improved biocompatibility. Further studies investigating inflammatory responses, such as laser flare photometry in IPCL patients, and inclusion of larger cohort groups are needed for a more comprehensive comparison of Collamer and IPCL biocompatibility profiles.

Supplementary Materials: The following supporting information can be downloaded at https://www.mdpi.com/article/10.3390/medicina61081384/s1, Table S1. Number of lenses used per treatment group.

Author Contributions: Conceptualization, K.I. (Kei Ichikawa), Y.T. and N.Y.; methodology, K.I. (Kei Ichikawa), Y.T., R.H., Y.K. and N.Y.; software, Y.T.; validation, K.I. (Kei Ichikawa), Y.T., Y.K. and N.Y.; formal analysis, N.Y.; investigation, K.I. (Kei Ichikawa); resources, R.H. and K.I. (Kazuo Ichikawa); data curation, Y.K. and N.Y.; writing (original draft preparation), K.I. (Kei Ichikawa) and Y.T.; writing (review and editing), K.I. (Kazuo Ichikawa) and N.Y.; visualization, Y.K. and N.Y.; supervision, K.I. (Kazuo Ichikawa); project administration, K.I. (Kazuo Ichikawa) and N.Y.; funding acquisition, K.I. (Kazuo Ichikawa). All authors have read and agreed to the published version of the manuscript.

Funding: This research received no external funding.

Institutional Review Board Statement: This study was conducted in accordance with the Declaration of Helsinki, and approved by the Chukyo Eye Clinic Ethics Committee (protocol code: No. 20250519095 and date of approval: 19 May 2025).

Informed Consent Statement: This retrospective study was approved by Chukyo Eye Clinic Ethics Committee (No. 20250519095) and adhered to the tenets of the Declaration of Helsinki. Due to the retrospective design, the Ethics Committee approved an opt-out method for including patient data to maintain anonymity instead of requiring written informed consent, which had been obtained for the original operations.

Data Availability Statement: The dataset is available from the authors upon reasonable request.

Acknowledgments: The authors are indebted to Masato Morikawa for editing and reviewing this manuscript for English language and technical support, and to David Price for English proofreading.

Conflicts of Interest: The funders (STAAR Surgical Co.) had no role in the design of this study; in the collection, analyses, or interpretation of data; in the writing of the manuscript; or in the decision to publish the results.

Abbreviations

The following abbreviations are used in this manuscript:

FN	Fibronectin
HEMA	Hydroxyethyl Methacrylate
ICL	Implantable Contact Lens
iHIE-NY2	immortalized human iris epithelial cells
IOL	Intraocular lens
IPCL	Implantable Phakic Contact Lens
PHAKIC-ICL	Phakic Implantable Contact Lens
WST-8	2-(2-methoxy-4-nitrophenyl)-3-(4-nitrophenyl)-5-(2,4-disulfophenyl)-2H-tetrazolium, monosodium salt
SD	Standard deviation

References

1. Munnerlyn, C.R.; Koons, S.J.; Marshall, J. Photorefractive keratectomy: A technique for laser refractive surgery. *J. Cataract Refract. Surg.* **1988**, *14*, 46–52. [CrossRef]
2. Pallikaris, L.G.; Papatzanaki, M.E.; Stathi, E.Z.; Frenschock, O.; Georgiadis, A. Laser in situ keratomileusis. *Lasers Surg. Med.* **1990**, *10*, 463–468. [CrossRef]
3. Sachdev, G.; Ramamurthy, D. Long-term safety of posterior chamber implantable phakic contact lens for the correction of myopia. *Clin. Ophthalmol.* **2019**, *13*, 137–142. [CrossRef]
4. Taneri, S.; Oehler, S.; Heinz, C. Inflammatory response in the anterior chamber after implantation of an angle-supported lens in phakic myopic eyes. *J. Ophthalmol.* **2014**, *2014*, 923691. [CrossRef] [PubMed]
5. Ichikawa, K.; Ichikawa, K.; Yamamoto, N.; Horai, R. Flexural and cell adhesion characteristic of phakic implantable lenses. *Medicina* **2023**, *59*, 1282. [CrossRef]
6. Lovisolo, C.F.; Reinstein, D.Z. Phakic intraocular lenses. *Surv. Ophthalmol.* **2005**, *50*, 549–587. [CrossRef] [PubMed]

7. Bhandari, V.; Karandikar, S.; Reddy, J.K.; Relekar, K. Implantable collamer lens V4b and V4c for correction of high myopia. *J Curr Ophthalmol* **2015**, *27*, 76–81. [CrossRef] [PubMed]
8. Klebe, R.J.; Bentley, K.L.; Schoen, R.C. Adhesive substrates for fibronectin. *J. Cell Physiol.* **1981**, *109*, 481–488. [CrossRef] [PubMed]
9. Hosny, M.H.; Shalaby, A.M. Visian implantable contact lens versus AcrySof Cachet phakic intraocular lenses: Comparison of aberrmetric profiles. *Clin. Ophthalmol.* **2013**, *7*, 1477–1486. [CrossRef]
10. Hong, Y.; Xin, J.; Wang, P.; Song, Y.; Fan, X.; Yang, L.; Guo, G.; Fu, D.; Dai, Y.; Zhang, F.; et al. Enhancing the biocompatibility of phakic intraocular lens via selective fibronectin trapping. *Acta Biomater.* **2025**, *197*, 240–255. [CrossRef]
11. Sanders, D.R.; ICL in Treatment of Myopia (ITM) Study Group. Postoperative inflammation after implantation of the implantable contact lens. *Ophthalmology* **2003**, *110*, 2335–2341. [CrossRef]
12. Tamada, Y.; Ikada, Y. Effect of preadsorbed proteins on cell adhesion to polymer surfaces. *J. Colloid Interface Sci.* **1993**, *155*, 334–339. [CrossRef]
13. Yamamoto, N.; Takeda, S.; Hatsusaka, N.; Hiramatsu, N.; Nagai, N.; Deguchi, S.; Nakazawa, Y.; Takata, T.; Kodera, S.; Hirata, A.; et al. Effect of a lens protein in low-temperature culture of novel immortalized human lens epithelial cells (iHLEC-NY2). *Cells* **2020**, *9*, 2670. [CrossRef]
14. Yamamoto, N.; Hiramatsu, N.; Ohkuma, M.; Hatsusaka, N.; Takeda, S.; Nagai, N.; Miyachi, E.I.; Kondo, M.; Imaizumi, K.; Horiguchi, M.; et al. Novel technique for retinal nerve cell regeneration with electrophysiological functions using human iris-derived iPS cells. *Cells* **2021**, *10*, 743. [CrossRef] [PubMed]
15. Guell, J.L.; Morral, M.; Kook, D.; Kohnen, T. Phakic intraocular lenses part 1: Historical overview, current models, selection criteria, and surgical techniques. *J. Cataract Refract. Surg.* **2010**, *36*, 1976–1993. [CrossRef] [PubMed]
16. Alfonso, J.F.; Baamonde, B.; Fernandez-Vega, L.; Fernandes, P.; Gonzalez-Meijome, J.M.; Montes-Mico, R. Posterior chamber collagen copolymer phakic intraocular lenses to correct myopia: Five-year follow-up. *J. Cataract Refract. Surg.* **2011**, *37*, 873–880. [CrossRef] [PubMed]
17. Zhang, Q.; Gong, D.; Li, K.; Dang, K.; Wang, Y.; Pan, C.; Yan, Z.; Yang, W. From inception to innovation: Bibliometric analysis of the evolution, hotspots, and trends in implantable collamer lens surgery research. *Front. Med.* **2024**, *11*, 1432780. [CrossRef]
18. Sechler, J.L.; Corbett, S.A.; Wenk, M.B.; Schwarzbauer, J.E. Modulation of cell-extracellular matrix interactions. *Ann. N. Y. Acad. Sci.* **1998**, *857*, 143–154. [CrossRef]
19. Gonzalez-Lopez, F.; Bilbao-Calabuig, R. Phakic intraocular lenses: Adapting to change. *Arch. Soc. Esp. Oftalmol. (Engl. Ed.)* **2020**, *95*, 157–158. [CrossRef]
20. Ofuji, K. Differential tyrosine phosphorylation of paxillin in human corneal epithelial cells on extracellular matrix proteins. *Jpn. J. Ophthalmol.* **2000**, *44*, 189. [CrossRef] [PubMed]
21. Altankov, G.; Groth, T. Fibronectin matrix formation by human fibroblasts on surfaces varying in wettability. *J. Biomater. Sci. Polym. Ed.* **1996**, *8*, 299–310. [CrossRef]
22. Zhu, A.; Zhang, M.; Wu, J.; Shen, J. Covalent immobilization of chitosan/heparin complex with a photosensitive hetero-bifunctional crosslinking reagent on PLA surface. *Biomaterials* **2002**, *23*, 4657–4665. [CrossRef]
23. Guarnieri, D.; De Capua, A.; Ventre, M.; Borzacchiello, A.; Pedone, C.; Marasco, D.; Ruvo, M.; Netti, P.A. Covalently immobilized RGD gradient on PEG hydrogel scaffold influences cell migration parameters. *Acta Biomater.* **2010**, *6*, 2532–2539. [CrossRef]
24. Ross, R. Atherosclerosis--an inflammatory disease. *N. Engl. J. Med.* **1999**, *340*, 115–126. [CrossRef] [PubMed]
25. Esmon, C.T. The interactions between inflammation and coagulation. *Br. J. Haematol.* **2005**, *131*, 417–430. [CrossRef] [PubMed]
26. Hung, H.S.; Tang, C.M.; Lin, C.H.; Lin, S.Z.; Chu, M.Y.; Sun, W.S.; Kao, W.C.; Hsien-Hsu, H.; Huang, C.Y.; Hsu, S.H. Biocompatibility and favorable response of mesenchymal stem cells on fibronectin-gold nanocomposites. *PLoS ONE* **2013**, *8*, e65738. [CrossRef] [PubMed]
27. Daum, R.; Mrsic, I.; Hutterer, J.; Junginger, A.; Hinderer, S.; Meixner, A.J.; Gauglitz, G.; Chasse, T.; Schenke-Layland, K. Fibronectin adsorption on oxygen plasma-treated polyurethane surfaces modulates endothelial cell response. *J. Mater. Chem. B* **2021**, *9*, 1647–1660. [CrossRef]
28. Cannas, M.; Denicolai, F.; Webb, L.X.; Gristina, A.G. Bioimplant surfaces: Binding of fibronectin and fibroblast adhesion. *J. Orthop. Res.* **1988**, *6*, 58–62. [CrossRef]
29. Schroeder, A.C.; Lingenfelder, C.; Seitz, B.; Grabowy, U.; WSpraul, C.; Gatzioufas, Z.; Herrmann, M. Impact of fibronectin on surface properties of intraocular lenses. *Graefes Arch. Clin. Exp. Ophthalmol.* **2009**, *247*, 1277–1283. [CrossRef]
30. Vesaluoma, M.; Mertaniemi, P.; Mannonen, S.; Lehto, I.; Uusitalo, R.; Sarna, S.; Tarkkanen, A.; Tervo, T. Cellular and plasma fibronectin in the aqueous humour of primary open-angle glaucoma, exfoliative glaucoma and cataract patients. *Eye* **1998**, *12 Pt 5*, 886–890. [CrossRef]

MDPI AG
Grosspeteranlage 5
4052 Basel
Switzerland
Tel.: +41 61 683 77 34

Medicina Editorial Office
E-mail: medicina@mdpi.com
www.mdpi.com/journal/medicina

www.ingramcontent.com/pod-product-compliance
Lightning Source LLC
Chambersburg PA
CBHW041954260926
51850CB00019B/2711
* 9 7 8 3 7 2 5 8 5 5 8 1 0 *